**What D**

Victoria Midwifery Group

Breathe n Believe!

*Kim Turton*

DEB LITTLE, R.M.
2000 Beach Drive
Victoria, B.C.  V8R 6J6
(250) 592-0099

# What Does a Doula Do?

Birth Coaching for an
Easy, Joyful, Loving Birth

## KIM TURTON

First Published in Great Britain 2011 by Influence Publishing
(an imprint of Bookshaker)

**Disclaimer**
This book was written for informational purposes only, to
encourage and educate pregnant mums and dads on the birth
choices for their babies. I use the reference to dads and partners
loosely, as I choose not to put labels on the mother's partner,
whether it is her boyfriend, husband or same sex partner. At the
same time, I also interchange the words boy and girl when
referring to the baby, while not specifically meaning either sex.

Please note I am not a professional medical authority. The
information in this book is intended to be used for general
information only, and should not replace consultation with
health care professionals. Always seek medical advice from
your own health care provider.

# Praise

"I get shivers of joy imagining other moms having this support in their birthing experiences, to have a doula journey with them - an experienced guide to travel the unknown terrain ... an amazing support for moms and their partners, offering them strength, wisdom and clarity of potential choices to support the child into the world all delivered in the caring and loving energy of the author."

**Canela Michelle Meyers, author of *Right Here, Right Now Meditations*, www.canelamichelle.com**

"A wonderfully thorough and comprehensive journey through everything that doulas provide for the pregnancy, birth and postpartum period. This book will help families prepare for their birth and make informed choices, including which doula would best suit their needs."

**Amanda Reid, RM & RN**

"This book demonstrates to us how we can choose to make our child's entrance into the world a celebration of the miraculous process that it is, instead of the clinical experience modern medicine has sometimes made it into. The birth stories that Kim has interspersed throughout the book really demonstrate how a birth coach empowers parents by providing them with education, tools and loving care during pregnancy, labour and delivery."

**Denise Cunningham, Bestselling author of *Whispers of Hope: Transcending Abuse, Cancer and Divorce to Embrace Peace*, www.journeyhome.ca**

*"Give this book as a shower gift. It contains an experienced doula's thoughts about how doulas can help women create an easier and happier birth experience. It covers a compendium of topics including: birth stories, ideas, birth notes by a doula, birth plans, breast-feeding, quotes, dads and doulas, doula techniques, postpartum services and common pregnancy, labor, birth and postpartum questions. Open this book and a wealth of information will spill out!"*

**Paulina (Polly) Perez, RN, BSN, FACCE, LCCE, CD author of *Special Women, Doula Programs* and *The Nurturing Touch at Birth***

## What Kim's Clients Say

*Kim was with us for the birth of both of our children, and we were so thankful both times to have her there. With our first son Fraser, we didn't know what to expect – from labour, from a doula, from the nurses, from anything. Kim was our kind, experienced guide. She guided my husband with ideas of how to help me (both births were non-C-section). He wouldn't have really known what to do without her, and I was in no position to coach him with how to coach me. Kim also called on nurses and took charge in a few instances when we might not have had the gumption to get them in line.*

*Kim has a great energy. She is totally there for you, but not in your face in any way. She is calming but not sappy. She is knowledgeable and reassuring.*

*So the second time around we figured we knew what we were doing – who needs a doula? But we thought "just to be safe" we would engage Kim again. And we were so glad we did. Our daughter Holland came quite fast, as many seconds do, but without Kim telling me to relax and just let Holly do the work, the experience would not have been as "enjoyable" as it truly was. And that is saying something! Kim made labour enjoyable the second time around.*

**Andrea**

*I can't imagine going through the awesome birth experience we had without Kim. There are so many things to know having your first child, or rather so many things you feel you should know, and don't. Kim answered all our questions and kept me focused and calm through the pregnancy and birth process.*

*The birth of our child had some serious complications for both mother and child (we are all doing wonderful today) and my husband is very grateful that Kim was also there for him!*

*Kim was always available to chat with and was also very respectful and never "took over" and she ensured my husband was my #1 supporter. (But boy, he needed her support!) I had a long labour and although the nurses were great at the hospital, they just don't have the time to stay with you and guide you through the "management" of labour.*

*Thank goodness Kim was there to suggest so many techniques such as breathing and positions to help me through it. When you're in that moment, it is hard to think clearly and remember everything you're supposed to do. As I mentioned we did not have a "typical" labour and delivery, so my experience was very different than most. And these are things you can't anticipate. We are so happy that we had Kim there with us. Don't know how we would have done it without her.*

**Erin**

I had an amazing experience with Kim. After having my first two children in the UK, the first being a fairly traumatic birth experience and the second being a C-section as suggested by the medical team, I was certain I would just have another C-section with my third. I had many discussions with my doctor about the impending birth and was encouraged to try for a VBAC at BC Women's Hospital and Health Centre in Vancouver. I had used a doula once before and loved the idea of having someone with me throughout the labour and the birth who could not only provide me with the support I needed, but would also provide the same for my husband.

Kim provided exactly that from the moment I phoned to tell her I was being admitted, to the moment I was taken into theatre (following a gruelling 12-hour labour). Kim encouraged my husband with advice on how to support me and was a calm and reassuring presence throughout the labour. As a wonderful gesture a week or so following my daughter's birth, she visited us at home with her beautifully written account of the labour and birth, something I will treasure forever.

**Natasha**

Thank you so much for all your support – you helped me support my wife so well and kept me from panicking many times. We couldn't have imagined our experience without you! (Dad)

We want to say a huge THANK you for your support as we experienced welcoming our new baby girl into the world. Words aren't enough to describe how grateful we are that you were there. Your presence, energy, support and experience were so valuable in reaching our ultimate goal of the birth of our daughter. We honestly do not think we could have done it as well without you and we are thrilled to have had you as our doula to share the experience. (Mum)

**Anonymous Couple**

**For my Mum**
*You show me what it means to be a strong woman.*
*Thank you for encouraging me with your unconditional*
*love. You are truly my best friend.*
*I love you.*

*I thought my first birth would be a natural vaginal birth with my husband at my side. We had no knowledge of doulas. I use this book to introduce you to the benefits of doulas in the hopes that your birth experience is more joyous.*

## Birth

I WAS FINALLY WHEELED into the operating room. My husband was changing into surgical scrubs as I was lying on the stretcher in a cold, sterile room, and nurses were rushing around my head. Eventually, my husband was ushered in to sit beside me. We sat behind a large, green sheet hanging three inches in front of us. My arms were strapped down to prevent me from shaking too hard, while under the influence of the drugs used to numb me from the neck down. We could see nothing but each other and the green sheet. Within minutes, after the sensation of tugging at my belly, the doctor had pulled my 9 lb 15 oz son, with a large head, out of my body. The nurse placed him on my chest. I was vibrating so badly from the drugs, that I thought I would jiggle him off of me and onto the floor.

The next thing I remember was waking up two hours later in a dark recovery room, no husband and, most definitely, no baby! There was no skin-to-skin contact, no breast-feeding at birth. I had barely seen my baby before I fell into a total blackout sleep.

Later, when I woke up and after this insult, I was told I had to stay three more days in the hospital. My thoughts turned to my poor mum who was back at home waiting to look after me and my baby...

*We've all been waiting for you.*
*For you.*
*Your arrival has been marked, has been recorded*
*on earth,*
*in the universe,*
*in the galaxies,*
*in all of space,*
*in all of time.*
*You come with a birthright, written in love and sung*
*through all Creation in words which promise*
*that no matter where you're at,*
*you're home*
*that no matter who you're with,*
*you're welcome*
*that no matter who you are,*
*you're loved.*
*Welcome.*

**Rita Ramsey**

# Contents

# Acknowledgments

*"Speak tenderly to them. Let there be kindness in your face, in your eyes, in your smile, in the warmth of your greeting. Always have a cheerful smile. Don't only give your care, but give your heart as well."*
**Mother Teresa**

## Clients

I CAME UP WITH THE IDEA of this book after hearing so many mums tell me that they needed encouragement, not the negative and disturbing birth stories that are so prevalent. So I thank all of those people for asking. I have written this book for you and for all the other pregnant couples seeking to have a fabulous birth.

I am so grateful to my clients for allowing me to use their birth stories and baby pictures in this publication. This gift is beyond generous.

The stories are all true. The women that I have written about, just like every other woman I help through the birthing process, prove to me that women are strong and determined. We contort our bodies and breathe through the most unbelievable marathon each time we birth our babies. Our inspiration and prize is the baby we birth, and the outcome is so incredibly worth our efforts.

Over the last ten years I have been so blessed to have amazing, warm and generous clients that have invited me to be their doula. I am honoured to have been able to help you on your journey through your personal, magical birthing moments. You make it easy for me to love my passion of birth.

## Family and Friends

I thank my partner in crime, Kim P, for being so amazingly generous, with your love and understanding. Even on vacation you never once complained that I might be spending too much time writing. – Love you!

When I started this labour of love Kim Tebbutt, my Reiki Master, stepped up and became my Angel. She spoke her wise words, used her warm heart along with comforting guidance to help me navigate this book to completion. What a blessing you are, my friend.

I belong to a wonderful group of authors that have published and will be publishing their books soon. The Spiritual Author's and Inspired Author's groups, you are amazing and talented groups of men and women that have helped me *birth* my book. I look forward to reading yours soon.

Warm thanks to Denise Cunningham, author of *Whispers of Hope, Transcending Abuse, Cancer and Divorce to Embrace Peace,* for guiding me so eloquently. You are truly a generous soul.

Linda Sajiw, a soon to be author, thank you for always finding fabulous resources for me.

Jessica Krippendorf Kirby, my editor extraordinaire, you pulled me out of a crunch and are brilliant at making my words very readable.

Julie Salisbury, my fairy publisher, sprinkling and throwing your magic all around so I can speak to the world.

PC for always wanting to help at my births.

# Labour

Dictionary.com defines labour as:

- Physical or mental work, esp. of a hard or fatiguing kind; toil.
- A job or task done or to be done.
- The physical effort and periodic uterine contractions of childbirth. The interval from the onset of these contractions to childbirth.

## Doula

According to Wikipedia, doula is a word that has most closely become associated with a woman, or man who provides non-medical support to other women and their families during labour and childbirth, and also during the postpartum period.

# Foreword

THERE WAS A TIME WHEN I would never have summoned up the courage to introduce you to Kim Turton's informative book about doulas. Having been assigned my biological package well before the doctor pronounced that I was indeed a "boy", I spent my early adult life believing that the mysteries of pregnancy and birth were matters best left to women and their medical consultants. While working as a child psychologist and therapist, I made the convenient assumption that babies only become real people when they begin to think rationally – somewhere around the age of three. Before that they were ... well ... you know ... babies.

Over the past thirty years my beliefs have changed radically. Like every other human being, I actually know a lot about life in the womb and the epic journey we must take down the birth canal and out into the great unknown. Throughout this critical phase of life, my mother was my constant provider and companion but, without me, it would have been a meaningless exercise. In other words, she and I were in this thing together from the get-go, facing the many challenges nature has created in bringing new life into the world. I now believe that birth – the passage from the security of the womb to the unpredictability of the outside world – may well be our most foundational developmental experience.

If you think this is a romantic notion, please think again. Research in the field of pre- and perinatal psychology clearly shows how mothers and their babies communicate from conception onwards through neuro-hormonal pathways embedded in the placenta (the only human organ actually shared by two people). Through the second trimester of the pregnancy, the unborn child is not only responding to Mom's emotions and thoughts, but is becoming increasingly aware of events taking place in the outside world. So by the time the infant makes that first eye-to-eye contact with Dad, or Mother's partner, their relationship is already established. In other words, babies come into this world as conscious, purposeful and relational beings. Within the natural order, birth is a crisis in our most primary relationship and what happens through this physical and emotional separation has profound and life-long implications for both mother and child.

In spite of this evidence, our culture continues to regard birth as a medical event in which the mother is a patient and the child a foreign object to be removed – a surgical procedure known as a "delivery". In true medical fashion the emphasis is upon the mechanics of operation with little or no attention being given to the relational aspects of the drama unfolding in the birthing room. A "successful" delivery is one that follows the prescribed medical protocols regardless of the physical or emotional trauma being experienced by the two central protagonists. It's worth noting that, in the 1930s, the eminent psychiatrist Otto Rank concluded that virtually all adult mental health problems could be traced back to unrecognized birth traumas. His colleague Sigmund Freud firmly agreed and declared this to be the most significant progress since the discovery of psychoanalysis.

Enter the doula. Here is a professional birth-specialist who operates beyond the mechanics of medical practice to create a special relationship from which mother can be fully connected with her baby throughout this pivotal and transformational event. By supporting mom through her many challenges, drawing dad (or mother's partner) into the action and inviting significant others to participate, a doula can turn a birthing procedure into a shared celebratory occasion. My personal and professional experience over the past fifty years has left me in no doubt that children who are welcomed into the world in this way are presented with a gift that will last a lifetime. On the other hand, children who are surgically induced into a sterile environment with a mother absent through fear or medication begin their journey in a very different way.

Enter Kim Turton. Here is an experienced doula offering a practical, down-to-earth guide for parents and prospective parents who understand that every child deserves a welcoming committee. Rich in thoughtful observations, personal insights and birth stories this book is a delightful introduction to birthing in its most wonderful and humane form. In her unassuming way, Kim Turton obviously believes that the doula's contribution can bring life and wonder back into the miracle of birth. I happen to believe that the methods she advocates can change the world.

**Gerry Fewster, Ph.D**
**author of *Don't Let Your Kids Be Normal:***
***A Partnership for a Different World***

# Introduction

IN MY BUSY DOULA PRACTICE, I am constantly being asked questions. The one I hear the most is, "Where can I find good positive birth stories? I can't seem to find any."

Women are trying to educate themselves about the natural birth process via the Internet, television, prenatal classes and other books. Being able to read accounts of births where there is ease and success is important. If women only find stories that are negative and involve long gruelling scenarios, it increases their anxiety for their impending birth, and that can lead to complications.

We have all heard stories from our friends and family about how long and hard their labour was, and how some had to have drugs, serious interventions and possibly Cesarean sections. *This does not have to be the norm.* When you have a doula helping you and your partner during your labour, you are allowing for a more positive outcome at birth.

In my practice, I write a birth story for my private clients about their labour and birth, and then present them with their story at the postpartum visit. With my clients' permission, I have taken their real birth stories and am presenting them in this book for all to enjoy. My goal is to help you realize that birth can be achieved with little or no use of drugs, whether you are in the home or hospital or are using a doctor, obstetrician or midwife.

I will explain some of the services a doula provides, how to find a doula and questions to ask during the interview process. In addition, you'll learn what to take to the hospital, how to be better prepared for labour and what it will look like, breast-feeding tips and what to expect once you get home. I also have a section of commonly asked questions by first-time and multiple birth parents, and a section where new parents give some fascinating tips for when you get home with baby.

When a woman is comfortable with the expectations of labour and most of the mystery is taken away, she can have a wonderful labour and birth. With the guidance of a doula, you can make a huge difference in your overall experience. I hope you enjoy these real birth stories from women just like you.

## Doula Statistics

Statistics have proven that doulas make a huge impact on the comfort of a labouring woman by helping her to achieve an easier, quicker birth. These numbers continue to increase as doulas become more popular and attend more births. It makes perfect sense to have help during this time when you are so involved in just trying to breathe.

It is a required medical procedure to have your care provider, whether a doctor, midwife or obstetrician, at your birth. It should also be essential to have a doula, as doulas can be an integral part of creating a positive birthing experience.

Klaus, Kennell, and Klaus (1993) compiled the results of over fifteen years work with over 1,500 women from several different countries in *Mothering the Mother: How a Doula Can Help You Have a Shorter Easier and Healthier Birth*. According to the authors, the benefits of using a doula are as follows:

- 50% reduction in Cesarean rates
- 25% shorter labour
- 60% reduction in epidural requests
- 40% reduction in syntocinon (Oxytocin) use
- 30% reduction in analgesia use
- 40% reduction in forceps delivery

*"If a doula were a drug, it would
be unethical not to use it."*
**John H. Kennell**

## Continuous Support for Women During Childbirth

This is a Cochrane review abstract and plain language summary, prepared and maintained by The Cochrane Collaboration.

*Continuous support in labour increased the chance of a spontaneous vaginal birth, had no harm, and women were more satisfied.*

*Historically women have been attended and supported by other women during labour and birth. However in many countries, as more women are giving birth in hospital rather than at home, continuous support during labour has become the exception rather than the norm. This may contribute to the dehumanization of women's childbirth experiences. Modern obstetric care frequently subjects women to institutional routines, which may have adverse effects on the progress of labour. Supportive care during labour may involve emotional support, comfort measures, information and advocacy. These may enhance physiologic labour processes as well as women's feelings of control and competence, and thus reduce the need for obstetric intervention. The review of studies included 21 trials, from 15 countries, involving more than 15,000 women in a wide range of settings and circumstances. The continuous support was provided either by hospital staff (such as nurses or midwives), women who were not hospital employees and had no personal relationship to the labouring woman (such as doulas or women who were provided with a modest amount of guidance), or by companions of the woman's choice from her social network (such as her husband, partner, mother, or friend). Women who received continuous labour support were more likely to give birth 'spontaneously', i.e. give birth with neither caesarean nor vacuum nor forceps. In addition, women were less likely to use pain medications, were more likely to be satisfied, and had slightly shorter labours. Their babies were less likely to have low 5-minute Apgar Scores. No adverse effects were identified. We conclude that all women should have continuous support during labour. Continuous support from a person who is present solely to provide support, is not a member of the woman's social network, is experienced in providing labour support, and has at least a modest amount of training, appears to be most beneficial. Support from a chosen family member or friend appears to increase women's satisfaction with their childbearing experience.*

# 1. Birth: My Story

I LOVED BEING PREGNANT ... all four times. I was always so excited when I missed my first cycle. I would buy pregnancy tests and take them too soon, only to receive a negative result. I would then have to go out, buy another one and wait. I loved watching for my stomach to grow and waiting patiently for the first flutters of movement at 20 weeks—the magical halfway mark.

Of course, some people hate being pregnant and are more than willing to speak negatively about their pregnancy stories. I will admit that the morning sickness, especially with my first son, was bad. But, it didn't come close to what some of my clients have experienced. Some have had such bad morning sickness that they had to resort to prescription medication and *still* were unable to leave the house, go to work or enjoy any part of their day. I remember not feeling well enough to eat, but I knew that I had to. I would consume copious amounts of soda crackers or have ice cream with lots of fruit on top.

## The Due Date

The part that I didn't like about being pregnant was that I was at least ten days overdue with all four boys. There was no way to entice them out any earlier and I would not resort to taking castor oil. One night, as I was relaxing in the tub pregnant with my fourth son, I had convinced myself that this one would not be late like the last three. This one would be born on time. But not a chance; my body just liked to gestate for those extra days.

I prefer to tell my clients that the date doesn't matter. It only causes you to fret if you are overdue. I believe doctors and midwives should round the due date to a time of the month, such as beginning, middle or end. There are so many reasons that the forty-week marker and due dates can be inaccurate. However, because women can have irregular menstrual periods and can ovulate at different times during their cycles, this can create false due dates.

These measurements are then compared to the *average* of other babies at the same gestation week. This is what either confirms or adjusts your due date. This technique is not exact science and is quite often wrong. Other reasons it may be hard to get an exact measurement could be that the baby is squirmy in utero or that the ultrasound is not very clear.

My first birth was a long, two-day process. I had called my mum on the first day to tell her that I was in labour and had been since 5 a.m. She grabbed her belongings, got in her car and drove six and a half hours to get to me. When she arrived in the afternoon, I still was not in active labour. At 6 p.m., my husband and I said goodbye to my mum and left for the hospital. I felt that I had been labouring for so long. I was uncomfortable, tired and wanted some help other than what my husband could offer. This would have been the perfect time for a doula; but, I would not know about doulas for another nineteen years. This is not to say they were not practicing in my city, just that I had no knowledge of them.

After arriving at the hospital, the nurses checked my cervix and told us that I wasn't "that far along" and that I needed to walk the halls. I was only a couple of centimetres dilated but we were admitted anyway. Today, standard procedure is, if you aren't four to five centimetres, you get sent home. It makes perfect sense to go where you are comfortable and can labour in a familiar place. They usually offer a shot of Morphine in your rear and tell you to go home and sleep. I wish I would have had that option, but this was back in 1982 and so it was not the case.

A brand new women's hospital was supposed to open the month I was having my first son. Unfortunately, the opening was delayed, so that meant I had to be admitted to the hospital that, I swear, was built a hundred years prior. The walls in the hall were green, old and sterile. I hated walking them but I was afraid to go back into the room with the emotionally distant nurse, who probably should have told us to go home, but didn't. I can't remember anything else about that night or if I even slept. It's all a blur.

I do remember having a nurse come in around noon the next day to ask me if a resident doctor could come in to check me for dilation. I said, "Sure." Five minutes later, the doctor walked in. He was the spitting image of a friend of mine, down to the Wallabee shoes he wore. "My God!" I thought. I was so convinced that he *was* my friend that I could barely open my legs for him to check me. He must have thought I was crazy.

The cervical check indicated that I wasn't as dilated as they had hoped for but I did get offered an epidural, and was told that I should have a Cesarean section. I said an immediate, "Yes" to both. I was booked for a 3:00 p.m. C-section. The anaesthesiologist was promptly called in to give me my "epi." Relief was now on its way; or so I thought. I didn't know what I was in for.

At 3:30 p.m., the doctor came in to say that I was being bumped for an emergency C-section. At that point, I was feeling like I *was* an emergency. I was cranky, exhausted and had no idea of what was happening to me. My poor husband was no wiser. We simply weren't prepared for anything that we were actually going through. Having an advocate with us to tell us what was going on, and what was going to happen, would have been helpful.

Close to 5:30 p.m., the doctor came in to top-up my epidural and tell me it would soon be my turn for the Cesarean. So much for my having a natural birth. Instead, the experience was cold and sterile. My husband and I had taken the traditional prenatal classes together at our local community center but for some reason, we had missed the Cesarean section class. There was no mention of doulas back then.

Now, after all I had just gone through, I still had no idea what had happened to me. I was definitely disappointed about my circumstances, but at that point wanting to meet my baby was my only concern.

After three days of confinement in the hospital, I took my baby home, determined never to experience that again! Next time I would attempt a VBAC (vaginal birth after Cesarean.) I was so deflated and traumatized by the experience, but thankfully, Mother Nature and her healing ways took over. I quickly forgot the experience and plunged into breast-feeding and sleepless nights.

## Eight Years Later

I was pregnant with my second child, by my new husband, and I was not, under any circumstances, going to have a Cesarean again. I will always have that scar on my tummy and I will never forget that there was nothing pleasant about my first labour.

With this second pregnancy I did not have as much morning sickness, or maybe I just handled it better. It is a blessing being pregnant the second time because you know so much more and you aren't so worried. My vision for this next labour was more informed and I knew what I wanted. My second son was 8 lb, 7 oz and I delivered him vaginally. I distinctly remember this birth and the unique sensation after his head was delivered. He seemed so small compared to my first son. It felt as though he wiggled and rattled his way through the birth canal, just like a bag of bones.

## Three Years Later

When I arrived at hospital to deliver my third son, I was fortunate enough to get the only room downstairs that had a tub. As a VBAC I am always classified high-risk and am not able to go upstairs to the nice birthing suites. This labour was heavenly. I lounged in the tub until the nurse said, "Okay, we need you to get on the bed now." I said, "No way!" They forcibly removed me from the tub to lie on the bed with the head of my son presenting. I pushed a couple of times and the head was delivered. Then the doctor looked at me and said, "You have to push the shoulders." A couple of pushes later, my 10 lb, 1 oz son was born. Except for the shoulder part, this was a fabulous birth.

## Two Years After That

Two years later, on a lovely September day, my mum, who always came to town when I was having my babies, came with me to my 10:00 a.m. doctor's appointment. I loved the help and the company my mum provided for me and my babies. I was pleasantly surprised when my doctor informed me that I was already 5 cm dilated. I was surprised because I hadn't really felt any contractions yet. I don't know if it was the nice summer day or my mum's company, but either way, I was thrilled. I asked my obstetrician if it would be alright if I went for lunch, and he said, "Yes. Of course."

While at lunch with my mum, I started feeling some mild contractions. I told her that I wouldn't mind going to the hospital after we eat because I think maybe I'm ready to deliver. We arrived at the hospital around 1:00 p.m. and I was given a room. I told my mum that I should call my husband. She called him for me and then asked if she should go, once he arrived. I told her she could stay. Little did I know, she had always wanted to be invited to my births, but never said anything, and modesty had prevented me from asking her to attend. Silly me!

At 3:50 p.m., I gently delivered my fourth son into the world, with my mum guiding and watching me. He was 9 lb, 6 oz. I have always regretted not having my mum there for the other births. She gave me a calm I had never experienced with my other labours. Honestly, my mum turned out to be more of a coach with her voice and touch, than either of my husbands. She was my doula. "Wow," I thought, "having babies is easy."

I do love birth and I have learned to love every single part of the labour process.

## A Very Interesting Concept

I was fortunate to have met a gifted spiritual singer at an event. Her name is Denise Hagan. She is a wisp of a woman—tall, with a beautiful Irish accent. Denise's sense of humour is as cheeky as you would expect from a woman who is an Indigo Elemental. An indigo person is described as being empathetic, curious, strong-willed and independent. An elemental is someone who is warm, playful and loves entertaining. They tend to look like larger versions of fairies.

Denise is all of the above but her most amazing attribute is her voice. Denise is a petite woman but when she sings, strong, bold, angelic tones come through and I was totally mesmerised while listening to her.

After her performance, we talked and I told her what I do as a doula. Denise was totally fascinated and explained to me that the spirits that guide her had told her a story about what happens at birth. She said that the soul of the mother reaches up to the unborn baby's soul and attaches itself. The mother then guides that soul to her baby, who is waiting patiently to be born. When this attachment happens, then the labour can begin. How utterly magical, to think that the new mum unconsciously initiates this special event.

*"Only with trust, faith, and support can the woman allow the birth experience to enlighten and empower her. Women's strongest feelings, in terms of their birthings, positive and negative, focus on the way they were treated by their caregivers."*
**Annie Kennedy & Penny Simkin**

## My Definition of Doula

"Doula" has many meanings. I like to think that a doula, when asked to attend a birth, complements the team helping a woman deliver her baby. I am hired to help mum breathe and relax, allowing for her beautifully designed body to work efficiently and for the baby to make its descent through the birth canal, all the while appreciating that this is mum and dad's journey. I help dad to fully experience the birth at his comfort level, and to encourage him to help his wife as their baby is born.

I am with the couple for many hours leading up to the birth, reminding mum to breathe, and allowing her body to birth, making sure she is well-hydrated and that she is moving her body in the correct way to help baby move and make its way with as few interventions as possible.

The request for a natural birth is usually standard from all my clients but has a very different meaning for each different couple – essentially if they can have a vaginal birth without any or very few drugs, in a reasonable time frame, they are going to be happy. This may sound simplistic but with the help from a doula you can achieve a natural birth with more confidence and greater success.

There are so many different techniques a doula brings to a birth. Each doula brings her unique set of talents and techniques based upon her specific training and beliefs. I will try and cover most of the techniques used, which is by far not all that a doula will offer you. Please see chapter three for a lengthy list.

I am essentially a servant to the labouring woman for the birth process, and quite happily so. My confirmation that I have succeeded in my services is when at the end of a birth a mum can look at me and tell me that "I couldn't have done it without your help," or my favourite, "You are my Birth Angel." My work is extremely rewarding.

## Why I Became a Doula

The morning after my niece was born, we went to the hospital to visit. My brother Jon and his wife Nicola were in their postpartum room. We talked about how Nicola's friend, a doula, had helped her navigate through her labour. When Nicola felt out of control, the doula kept her focused and calm. Jon felt good that his task was to be the waiter. His main job was to get the ice, the water and the towels. Easy! Having a doula was good for both of them. Nicola was happy to have her dear friend attend the birth, and Jon was more than pleased to have the wisdom and talents of their friend. They both raved that having a doula was definitely the way to birth.

We talked more about the baby and the experience, and then I signed the visitor's book that they had brought for guests to sign. I loved the idea that family and friends had a place to write their first thoughts and comments about the new baby. I also loved the idea that a job existed where someone could help a woman in labour. I changed my career path that day. I knew there was going to be a lot more to learn, but I loved the fact that I would be able to attend a birth each day I worked.

## My Training

I love the concept of asking the Universe for help. I asked for, and received, all the information on doulas that I needed. At home, I quickly got on my computer, looked up the spelling of *doula*, and before I knew it, I was enrolled in the next course available at my local college. Only two doula classes were being offered each year. I started my class just three weeks after my niece was born. I would go to my current job, visualizing how wonderful it was going to be to get paid to watch babies being born.

Since then, I have had more training, which has helped me to excel in my profession. I took an extended breast-feeding course from *La Leche League International* because it is important for me to educate women about the importance of breast-feeding and what to do if they can't. Both mums and babies learn to breast-feed at birth. Sometimes it's not easy but with lots of encouragement, they can succeed. As a doula, I help educate women on this subject before they go into labour and after they have given birth.

I offer private prenatal classes to my clients. I've taken the *Lamaze Prenatal Educator Course*, which is probably the best-known prenatal course in Canada, and I've studied *Birthing from Within* written by Pam England and Rob Horowitz, and *HypnoBirthing - The Mongan Method* by Marie F. Mongan. All of these techniques offer fabulous ideas. I try to answer any questions that couples have regarding all aspects of birth, but I also refer them to specialists when needed.

In addition, I've trained with hypno-therapist Di Cherry, who has had a busy practice in Vancouver for many years. Part of her practice is helping women move through their fears in labour and delivery. This method, along with *how* you talk to women during labour, can make a huge difference.

I believe visualisation in labour has remarkable results and helps the mum to relax. Marie Mongan has great affirmations in her book, which also includes a meditation CD. You can look in any bookstore or on the Internet to find books and other CDs about visualization, meditation and music specific to labour and birth.

---

*A nice addition to the visualisation technique is to put sticky notes with positive affirmations all around the house – on the fridge, on mirrors, any place that you will easily notice them. I make up sayings while listening to my client at her prenatal visit. She'll tell me what she is concerned or anxious about and then I may suggest affirmations such as: I am a strong woman – I will easily birth this baby – Labour will be short and easy – My body is designed to birth with ease – or, as simple as, I can do it and Breathe and Believe. Choose anything that works best for you.*

---

My studies continue, inside and out of the labour and delivery room. I learn something new every day that I go to work. Birth is never the same and because of that, it makes my job more exciting and stimulating.

## How This Has Empowered Me

At the beginning of my career, I believed I had a small amount of control over someone's labour and delivery. My mind had the crazy idea that *I* was helping to achieve the perfect birth for this couple. I have seen so many different birthing scenarios and I am so humbled by my profession. I have been granted the gift of inclusion in very personal, life transforming moments of other people's lives. I encourage the labouring woman in front of me, and help her work to her full capacity of achieving a natural birth, this time knowing full well I have no control.

I am honoured to attend and assist with birth. This has contributed to my growth as a woman and to my becoming a better doula. I have glorious visions of being the best doula ever for my clients. This makes me push further to provide for each mum, while understanding that anything is possible in labour. I delight in the knowledge that Mother Nature and the will of "Spirit" or "Soul" is entering the body of the baby and is controlling the whole event, in perfection of the Divine's desires.

I have seen such strength in a woman when she is pushing, after she has been labouring for a long time, and then I've seen her soften her focus and position herself so the baby is on her chest, ready to breast-feed.

Tenacity – Strength – Will – Drive ... I could go on about what women are made of. I get to see this every day when I go to "work." It is easier to explain to people that I go to work, or my job, but I really go to my passion every day. I am blessed in my work. It helps me to be my best every single day and I strive to give the best service to my clients.

My compassion for people has grown as I've looked after my clients and their babies, and have interacted with the doctors, nurses, specialists, family and friends of the birthing couple. I continue to be a healer, teacher, author and spiritual provider, and to inspire others as much as I have been inspired.

> *"Attending births is like growing roses.*
> *You have to marvel at the ones that*
> *just open up and bloom at the first*
> *kiss of the sun but you wouldn't*
> *dream of pulling open the petal of the*
> *tightly closed buds and forcing them*
> *to blossom to your time line."*
> **Gloria Lemay**

## Danielle and Reggie's Birth Story

Sometimes, there is neither rhyme nor reason why a petite woman should have a baby so quickly with what seems like little effort and within a short time frame. My cousin was a woman like this and she almost didn't make it to the hospital. She has a slight build and her babies were all delivered within several hours. It truly makes you wonder how the pelvis opens so easily for some women and not so easily for others.

Another woman like this is Danielle, a woman in her 20s. Danielle is extremely passionate about life, expresses herself well and is open-minded and spiritual.

She and her husband Reggie are from a Southern town in the U.S. They were in Vancouver to work for the 2010 Winter Olympics. Danielle was hoping that the baby wouldn't be born on her and Reggie's first anniversary, which was two days after the baby's due date.

*Danielle and I have a fabulous prenatal visit where she describes to me what her natural labour would look like. Both "grandmas-to-be" were to be in the labour and delivery room with her and Reggie. Danielle is an actress so she's used to having her moves directed. Reggie's mother is going to be the videographer for the event. Danielle's aunt told her that all the children in the family came two weeks early so she knows this is a possibility for her as well. Danielle's mum is to arrive two weeks before the due date. The plan is set and everyone attending the birth knows what they are supposed to do. There is a lot of excitement for this birth.*

*Part of the plan is for a mirror to be in the room, so Danielle can watch the event. She is very interested in seeing the process of the birth in the moment. Reggie is going to catch their son and cut the cord. Danielle knows she can endure pain, and feels confident that little or no pain medication will be needed. She loves water and so she plans to labour in either the shower or a tub.*

*Reggie predicts that his son will be born three and a half weeks early, so it is no surprise when Danielle goes into labour at thirty-six and a half weeks. I get my first call from Reggie at 11:20 p.m. He says they have just returned from a movie after an enjoyable evening together, and Danielle's water has broken. Her contractions have started but are not regular yet. He wants to know what they should do. I advise Reggie that the care providers need to know what is happening and that they will advise him on the best way to make Danielle comfortable for the evening.*

*When water breaks in the middle of the night and there are no contractions, care providers will often advise mums to relax and try to get some sleep. I mention that Danielle can relax in a tub, drink some tea or warm milk and definitely try to sleep, even if it is just a nap. I explain that it will be a long night.*

*The next call from Reggie comes at 2:15 a.m. He tells me that Danielle's contractions are both regular and increasing in intensity. Since they are concerned, they decide to go to the hospital. They want to know if I will meet them there. I get dressed and jump into my car. The only good thing about getting out of bed at that time of the morning, and in the middle of winter, is that there is no traffic on the road. It is an easy drive to work.*

*By 2:50 a.m., the midwife comes into the assessment room, which is on the main level of the hospital, to check Danielle's cervix. She is 3 cm dilated and fully effaced. Danielle is managing well with each contraction. We are told that we can go upstairs to a room. We pack up their belongings and slowly set off toward the nicer delivery ward. The rooms upstairs in this hospital are newer and feel more like home. Actually, my clients refer to them as the hotel rooms. There are huge tubs in the middle of the rooms and the ability to set a variety of lighting scenarios so we can have a dimly lit and peaceful environment for baby's arrival.*

*It is 3:15 a.m. Reggie and I quickly put Danielle into the shower. She is breathing heavily and doing really well, but the frequency and intensity of contractions has increased and she needs instant relief. The shower helps her manage the pain that is getting stronger, while we run a tub.*

*The midwife has to leave to start the paperwork and order an I.V. set-up for the antibiotic drip. A nurse arrives to check on the room. She sees we have everything under control at the moment, so she leaves to set up Danielle's chart at the nurse's station.*

---

*Danielle needing an I.V. was part of the hospital protocol. Procedural testing for Group B streptococcus, or GBS, also known as Group B strep is done between weeks thirty-five and thirty-seven. If a woman tests positive, then antibiotics are administered in labour. If she tests negative, then it is not necessary. If labour starts before the care provider has received the test results, then protocol states that the antibiotic I.V. be administered.*

*Group B strep is bacteria found in the digestive and reproductive tracts of approximately 30% of women. If positive, the woman can potentially pass the bacteria to baby during labour, causing serious conditions like meningitis and sepsis, which can lead to blindness of the infant. All women are asked whether they tested positive or negative in the test when they are admitted to hospital.*

---

*3:30 a.m.: Within fifteen minutes, there are definite changes in Danielle's contractions. All of a sudden, she is asking for pain medications and her breath rate is increasing again. Now she is really showing signs of her body working hard. The shower is still working well and she sways her body in a dancing motion with each contraction. However, it is becoming more of an effort for Reggie and me to get her to control her breathing. The big contractions are coming back-to-back and are taking her breath away. She is almost panicking.*

*Five minutes later, Danielle says she can feel something coming out. I notice her involuntarily trying to push the baby. I motion for Reggie to get her out of the shower and bring her to the bed. I tell him I am going to get the midwife. I look at Danielle and urge her to breathe through the desire to push. It is very important not to push through the contractions.*

*I run out the door and down the hall. I find the midwife doing paperwork and quickly tell her what is going on. She grabs her papers. The nurse hears me from around the corner and calls for help on her portable phone. The three of us race into the room. I help Reggie get Danielle out of the shower. He hasn't gotten far in the 30 seconds that I was gone. We hold either side of Danielle, dry her and carry her to the bed, all within a fraction of a minute.*

*Everyone at the nursing station hears what is happening. The obstetrician and several nurses come running into the room. Two of the nurses are preparing the room for delivery while the obstetrician is trying to catch up with the midwife on Danielle's vitals and labour. The doctor puts on her gloves and motions to us to get Danielle onto the bed so she can check her cervix to see how she is really progressing.*

*Danielle is 10 cm dilated and ready to push. We help her turn around onto her hands and knees. She is determined to be upright, so she leans over the back of the bed. She looks at me with her big, beautiful, brown eyes and asks why it hurts so much. "Why are the pains coming so fast?" There is no other explanation than, "You're ready to push, Sweetie!"*

*3:39 a.m.: After only two very hard and huge pushes, a beautiful baby boy is born. Reggie helps to catch his son. The obstetrician grabs the baby and he is quickly taken to the bassinette where he is checked. He is perfect. His apgars are good. He is breathing well and crying, perfectly.*

*The apgar test is the first testing a baby has at birth. It's an acronym for **A**ppearance or skin colour, **P**ulse or heart rate, **G**rimace or reflex irritability, **A**ctivity or muscle tone, and **R**espiration. Scoring is 0 – 2 for each portion, with a total of 10 being perfect. The testing can be done while baby is on mum's chest. Usually, parents aren't even aware that the care providers are watching for these signs.*

*I help Danielle lay on the bed. There are several nurses scattered around the room, doing their duties – checking mum, checking baby, and helping the midwife. Total chaos!*

*The placenta is easily delivered at 3:45 am. Baby is monitored a while longer in the bassinette, because he was born a few weeks early. It was a quick birth and he was only 5 lbs. I can't believe the delivery took only nine minutes; shower to baby in nine minutes flat! Danielle watches everything happening in the room, amazed by the quickness of it all. I take out my camera to start taking pictures.*

*Danielle's son is finally brought to her. It's always an emotional moment when mum gets to meet her baby for the first time. Nine long months of waiting to see what he or she will look like, and then her life changes instantly. Every mum's reaction is subtly different but very magical, as you watch her fall in love with her new baby.*

*Danielle and Reggie spend a long time cuddling and getting to know their baby. Around 5:00 a.m., we put the baby to the breast, where he starts sucking almost immediately. He has a great latch and seems hungry from his quick slide into this new existence. I leave the room to prepare some toast and juice for mum. When I come back, I suggest that Reggie feed Danielle. I love it when a dad tenderly feeds the mother of his child, while she continues to nurse their baby.*

*At 6:00 a.m., mum and dad are getting tired and want to nap. They whisked their way through labour so quickly and it now it catches up with them. The room is finally quiet since all the nurses, the midwife and the obstetrician have left. I turn down the lights, set up the linens for the bed that dad will nap on and place baby in his bassinette. I hug the brand new parents and quietly take my leave.*

Unfortunately, there was no video-taped recording of the birth. No grandmas were called, because this baby was in such a hurry to arrive. Mum did a fabulous job managing all the contractions and she only asked for something to ease the pain when she was 10 cm and fully dilated. With ease and determination, she then pushed out her beautiful child into the world. Mum and dad had a bet with each other that dad would cry or shed a tear. He did neither, but I would have to say that he was bursting with pride as he watched his son being born.

Wow! Another day in paradise.

*Breathe and Believe.*

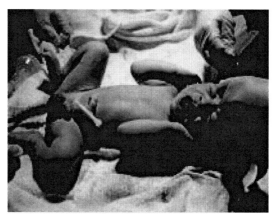

Baby being checked.

# 2. The South Community Birth Program

*"The whole point of woman-centered birth is the knowledge that a woman is the birth power source. She may need, and deserve, help, but in essence, she always had, currently has, and will have the power."*
**Heather McCue**

THE SOUTH COMMUNITY BIRTH PROGRAM is unique. I had heard about the program several years before joining. I was busy at the time with my private doula business – a single mum raising my children, and trying to work part-time at a grocery store. The combination was overwhelming and I couldn't think of adding more to my routine. Then at a meeting in September of 2009, four colleagues gave a presentation on the program and it inspired me to become a member of the team.

We work together as family, backing each other up in our doula work. I work with an extraordinary group of doctors and midwives that offer our pregnant couples complete and comprehensive prenatal, birth and postpartum care. The care providers show a passion for the work of delivering babies, and knowledge and compassion for the labouring mum. I am passionate about empowering women, and this program strives to empower women to be more independent and take better charge of their birth options.

The SCBP was established in the South Community of Vancouver, British Columbia. In December 2003 the office opened and the first baby was born in April 2004. The program's goal is to improve the health outcomes of low-risk pregnant women in the community of South Vancouver. It provides a unique collaborative program that includes family physicians, midwives, community health nurses and doulas.

This was the first such multidisciplinary program of its kind in Canada. Care takes place in a community-based, culturally appropriate and woman-centered manner during pregnancy, birth and the postpartum period. This initiative was set up to bring pregnancy and birth back to the community level and to improve the health outcome of women and their families.

Some of the goals developed by the SCBP are to set up an environment where we work with the families to meet their pre- and postnatal care needs in the community, allowing the couples to identify with their own strengths and build confidence in their ability to give birth and become parents. We support and encourage women and their families to assume a more active role in their own health care and help build a strong sense of peer support to encourage community and reduce the feeling of isolation.

The program encourages a safe, positive birth experience through the reduction of interventions, and post-delivery support, which allows women shorter hospital stays. When women play an active role in their care with proper education and are given the tools and skills to empower themselves in their pregnancies, they learn to better care for their babies. The feedback from the parents is that the group is highly effective and a satisfying way to receive care. The collaborative team of nurses, physicians, midwives and doulas has been a successful approach in reducing interventions, lowering rates of Cesarean sections, shortening the length of stay at hospital, and improving breast-feeding expectations.

When women come to SCBP the first few private appointments are for collecting personal history and physical exams. The women are asked if they would like to choose to go into a group setting. The group sessions start around week 18-20 of pregnancy, and include medical assessment, education and peer support, and bonding with the women that will later on be a support system as they raise their children in the same communities. The group includes women with due dates within a four-week period and includes a reunion night after all babies are born.

There are a total of ten sessions, and while at the appointment each woman weighs herself, takes her blood pressure and checks her urine. The care provider does the clinical tasks of checking uterine growth and listening to baby's heartbeat, called the "three-minute belly check." Each group is given a notebook that includes the material covered in the group discussion sessions. They are guided through birth preparation topics, and the group setting allows for questions and a chance to get to know other pregnant women living in the community. These women are making long-time friends for themselves and for their children.

Women who opt out of group sessions receive standard one-on-one care with a midwife or family physician for their routine prenatal care. Either program allows all the women to be attended in labour at BC Women's Hospital and Health Centre by the on-call midwife or family physician.

When necessary, women are referred to an obstetrician for a consultation or transfer of care. The SCBP providers function as a team, collaborating with community health nurses, doulas, dieticians, physiotherapists, social workers and translators, when necessary.

Jalana Grant CD (DONA), LCCE, is a certified labour doula with DONA International as well as a DONA International Approved Birth Doula Trainer. Jalana developed a multicultural doula program, including recruiting and training program doulas. She also established the system used for matching clients with their assigned doulas. She continues to recruit and maintain the doula and mentor teams, and supports both the doulas and the clients throughout their involvement with the program, ensuring a doula is available and in attendance during labour. She maintains a current database of available doulas, and is responsible for arranging the mentors and invoicing for doula services at the end of each month. She acts as a liaison between the doula team and program care providers, ensuring all aspects of the doula program run as smoothly as possible.

Jalana co-facilitates the Connecting Pregnancy sessions as do the program nurses. There is always a midwife or family physician and a co-facilitator at every Connecting Pregnancy group. The groups engage ten to twelve women through prenatal care and childbirth education. Each woman is offered a doula and very few choose not to have one. Jalana has each couple fill out a questionnaire to best place them with their doula.

The south Vancouver area community has a diverse multicultural population, so for most SCBP clients language and religious beliefs are important factors in choosing their doula. The program's doulas work to bring cultural competency and understanding to their clients' births.

SCBP can offer these women doulas that are speaking one of 26 different languages as well as English. The doulas have varied backgrounds and come from different countries; some were auxiliary nurses or midwives in their home country. Doulas, where possible, speak the client's first language. Some of the doulas act as a Cultural Broker by helping with translation at the clients' prenatal care visits, and aiding with communication with the hospital birthing staff.

Some doulas work in the community in a variety of other areas such as massage therapists and healing modalities like acupuncture and Reiki. Some are also school teachers, full-time mothers, professional translators and yoga instructors.

The care providers and some of the doulas attend the regular "meet the team" evenings for the couples. This is a friendly setting, where couples are given the opportunity to meet many of the team members, and are able to discuss questions about SCBP's role and how it will impact their labour.

The doulas meet with their clients once before the birth which gives both parties the chance to get to know each other and discuss any birth preferences the couple has. They next meet when the clients are in early labour and start the birthing journey. There may be telephone contact for several hours, or the doula is asked to come to the couple's home. Everything depends on what the woman feels and if she needs more support. Sometimes the call is to come to the hospital as the couple is going directly there.

Doulas stay with their clients for the labour, delivery and up to two hours postpartum, helping with breast-feeding. They also provide a postpartum visit to review the birth.

Doulas are on call 24/7 for the labouring woman and have a fabulous back-up doula network. There are some instances when doulas need to help one another, like when several clients birth within a couple of days. The doulas may be exhausted from a long birth, multiple clients go into labour on the same day or a doula is sick. There is always a doula at the birth (unless the client has declined one) as the concept is that the doula will be providing the continuity of care and support is always paramount.

SCBP's program is constantly growing and Jalana keeps the doulas busy. For more information on the SCBP please feel free to check out the website at *www.scbp.ca*.

Whether I work independently with a private client or Jalana assigns me a SCBP client, I love that I have such fabulous back-up help. Doulas work closely together. There should always be a back-up in case of emergency, and we have a large network of doulas we can draw from if needed.

*"For far too many women pregnancy and
birth is something that happens to them rather
than something they set out consciously
and joyfully to do themselves."*
**Sheila Kitzinger**

## When Back-up is Needed

My favourite story regarding my back-up was when my friend Michelle Maclean, another doula and a great friend, worked a crazy full moon weekend with me. It was July 11, 2010 – the eve of the New Moon Solar Eclipse. There was truly a mutual give and take that work day.

*The weekend starts with a call at 11:00 p.m. from Michelle. She has to wait for her husband to get home from work and asks if I can cover for her for several hours until she is able to attend to her client. I have just laid down for a nap and am waiting for my clients to call. They received Cervadil earlier in the day to induce labour, and are already in early labour.*

*I leave and go to Michelle's client's house. This woman is in fabulous labour with contractions coming often and strong. I am with her for several hours when she says she wants to go the hospital. The on-call care provider is with us at the home—this only happens if no other women are labouring at the hospital.*

*Michelle calls to say her husband is delayed. Can I stay? Yes! I advise her we are ready to go to hospital.*

*Meanwhile, my client, (we'll call her client A), is starting to have heavier contractions, and this concerns me. She is content at home and doesn't need me yet, so I carry on with Michelle's client (B).*

*At 6:00 a.m. Michelle is on her way to hospital, but with a different set of clients (client C). She is a multip— the couple is on their way in to hospital and having the baby now. The question again is, Can I stay longer with B? Again, I say Yes.*

---

A "multip" (slang) for Multipara refers to a woman who has delivered two or more babies. If the first was a vaginal delivery, multips usually have easier and faster births in subsequent deliveries.

A "primip" (slang) for Primipara refers to a woman who has delivered one baby.

A Multiple is when a woman is carrying more than one fetus in one pregnancy; twins, triplets or more.

---

*I have been with B for another hour when client A calls and says she needs me to come because the contractions are getting stronger. I call another back-up to be with client A for me.*

*At 7:00 a.m. client A calls and says they want to come to the hospital. Michelle is downstairs and the doctor is in the room with us, but has to run to catch the baby for clients C. Michelle will be busy for about another 1 ½ hours postpartum with her multip client C.*

*Client A has arrived at the hospital and is put in the assessment room to have her cervix checked. She is only 3 cm dilated. She was induced with Cervidil last night.*

*My back-up that is with client A is called at 8:30 a.m. to go to her clients. She asks if I have more back-up. Thank heavens Michelle is now free to see my client A in the assessment room.*

*Client A is given a shot of Morphine and sent home to try and nap, so Michelle quickly goes home to have a nap. I am with B upstairs and she is now pushing – I will be staying with these clients as I was the first doula on call. Keeping continuity for this labouring couple is paramount.*

*At 9:30 a.m. I quickly scoot out of the room to answer my phone. It's my client A, the one that had the Morphine shot, awake and wanting Michelle to come to their house, but they can't find Michelle's phone number. I relay the message to Michelle and quickly get back to my client who is getting ready to deliver*

*Poor Michelle barely has time to get home – I don't believe she has even rested – and goes to client A's house to help.*

*Client B has her baby, and I finally leave the room at 11:00 a.m. I go home to take a nap. But then I get a call at 2:15 p.m. and a progress report on client A. She is still 5 cm dilated and now they want to augment her contractions. Michelle will stay with them, but mentions another client (D), a multip, whose water has broken and may need me as back-up.*

*We text back and forth on our phones during the afternoon and into the evening. Michelle is still with client A and she is still 5 cm dilated. Michelle's client D has not progressed either, but she has to go by 5:00 a.m. tomorrow and will need back up—not to mention she hasn't slept. Michelle had been up 22 hours in the two days prior to when the craziness started.*

*The point I make here is that two girls are induced the same day – within half an hour of each other – both first time mums. One delivers in 15 hours, the other in 30 plus hours. Of the two girls that are multips, one delivers in three hours, the other in 12 hours and counting. It is now 9 p.m. with more babies to come. After I sneak in quick nap, I get the call to attend my next birth.*

Thank God Michelle is younger than me and has more stamina. It was total craziness. This was the start to my three births in four days, and by the end I couldn't remember my name

Consider how much time we, as doulas, give our clients: the phone calls and emails answered before, during and after birth; the time away from our families attending a birth can be 10 to 36 hours. We may stay the 36 hours or have someone relieve us briefly, as we take a quick nap or go home to shower. There are times we miss family activities, like birthdays or special family dinners and holidays. We accept this routine and lovingly get out of bed at 4:00 a.m. to race to a birth— even in the snow! When we do the math and figure out what we make on any individual birth, we really don't do this for the money, but for the pure joy.

*"Treating normal labors as though they were complicated can become a self-fulfilling prophecy."*
**Rooks**

## Doctors, Midwives and Doulas

Clients often ask, "Are doulas and midwives the same?" People confuse the two roles, which are distinctly different. Midwives and doulas are similar insofar as the care they give a client. Both tend to choose a more natural path to birth and methods for pain relief. Doulas work well *with* doctors and midwives; the care provider, and work *for* the mum and dad; the clients.

Doulas help educate couples through prenatal preparation, and we are with them during labour. We stay one to two hours following the birth, ensuring the baby can breast-feed and that the new parents are comfortable. Fees for visits and services are negotiable with some doulas, depending on the woman's needs. Doulas do not perform any clinical procedures.

Another common question is about the difference between doctors and midwives. The family can choose either for prenatal care, birth and postpartum care. Each would catch the baby and do all the clinical work.

From what I see in my community in Vancouver, there seems to have been a switch in primary prenatal care. Traditionally, care was provided by general practitioners or family physicians, with consultations made to specialists like obstetricians as required for high-risk issues. In British Columbia our medical system pays for either a doctor or a midwife; it is the family's choice who they want to attend the birth.

In my own pregnancies, I would see my general practitioner until I was in my third or fourth month and then transfer care to an obstetrician. This was because I had a Cesarean section with my first birth, and was then classified a high-risk pregnancy. When in labour it was my general practitioner that was called to help deliver my babies. I found the changing of practitioners to be disruptive for my prenatal care, but I had no other choice.

When doctors deliver babies, protocol is followed more closely; for example, medical procedures and medicines are offered a bit more readily in the process. The stress and strain of having a general office practice and the irregular hours of prenatal care make it difficult to provide care for all their patients. There are fewer general practitioners delivering babies than there were in the past. Mine chose to stop delivering babies, partly because of the work hours.

A complaint I commonly hear about attending doctor's appointments is that the appointment is quick, only fifteen minutes, and women wish they had more time to ask questions about their pregnancy and labour.

Today we see general practitioner doctors who are specializing in birth and work exclusively with pregnant women. These doctors are working in group clinics that provide similar philosophy and care. They have an on-call doctor that attends the birth which is done on a rotation basis.

The option to engage the services of a midwife has become more popular in the last ten years, and that increases with every birth they attend. They have privileges in the hospitals and they attend home births. There aren't as many midwives as people would like; because of high demand women have to engage midwifery services early in their pregnancy.

Midwives' training is specifically for low-risk and uncomplicated pregnancies, labour and postpartum care. They do not have a medical license so a midwife will refer a woman to a doctor or specialist if there are complications. She can not prescribe medicine or medical interventions.

Midwives do have training in homeopathic and natural healing techniques. For the most common pregnancy issues like morning sickness, induction of labour, management of labour pains and more, midwives take a natural approach, ensuring the health of mother and baby. When they attend home births, midwives always have a back-up plan in case problems with labour arise that are outside their general scope of practise.

Midwives work in clinics with other midwives and love prenatal and postpartum home visits, spending up to an hour per visit. The home visits include all of the regular checks that would otherwise occur at an office visit. During labour a midwife will attend a woman's home anytime, even in the middle of the night. She can assess dilation of the cervix, check baby's heart rate and the woman's temperature, and also help to make a plan if a woman needs help with the progression of labour. This helps avoid unnecessary hospital trips, and allows women to stay in the comfort of their homes for longer.

Midwives usually like to be present while you are labouring. They tend to be around more than doctors whether you are at home or hospital and they are more hands on with their suggestions for labour. Midwives catch your baby, and are open to having dad help catch your baby. Midwives can perform repair procedures as a doctor would if there are any tears or cuts to the vagina after birth.

## The Midwife and a Changed Birth Plan

*My client is in the care of a midwife. She phones me during the day to say she is in labour. Then later in the day she asks me to come over because she thinks things are progressing and she needs my help.*

*Minutes after I arrive, I ask dad if the midwife has been called. He says, "Yes, she was supposed to be on her way."*

*Five minutes later, after watching mum lean against the counter and move around, I can tell labour is progressing very quickly. There are some good signs that she might be further along than we all realize. I suggest dad call the midwife and tell her to come over right away.*

*With this encouragement the midwife drops what she is doing and comes over immediately.*

*The midwife examines my client, who is expecting to go to the hospital for the delivery. We find she is already 10 cm dilated. The midwife promptly asks her if she would like a home birth. Mum and dad have already decided they want a hospital birth, but everything changes in an instant.*

*We have a home birth and thank heavens it is a first birth. We have time to set things up quickly and put mum in the upstairs bedroom. We have her comfortable as can be in time for her baby. I am happy not to have to catch. If this had been a multip (second or third) I am sure I would have had to phone 911—after I caught her baby!*

## How the SCBP Makes a Difference in Community

You can easily go back more than one hundred years and read about small town living. I remember the small community I grew up in not far from Vancouver. There was such camaraderie where I went to school. I am still friends with a girl I met in grade five. My family knew all my neighbours very well, and I would babysit a younger boy down the street.

I don't see this any more. I don't know most of the people on my block. We have lost this close and friendly way of raising families. I certainly enjoy living in a big city now, but would love to see us return to a friendlier world.

I love to see that SCBP has made an impact on our clients' lives and is rebuilding a sense of community. As a society we are moving closer to a sustainable way of life, relying more heavily on living and buying in a hundred-mile radius, and working toward totally sustainable communities in which we can help each other as families and raise our children together.

SCBP birthing couples start this journey in their prenatal group, where friendships are made. My clients voluntarily tell me they are grateful that they are in the program. They are connecting with people that they will be sending their children to the same schools with in the future. But right now, they have a network of friends that can help each other as they birth their babies.

A perfect example of this closeness is when three of my couples bonded for life over their hospital stay. They were all from the same SCBP group, and all three women were admitted to hospital the same day. The next three days in a row they all delivered their babies, one day at a time.

While in hospital two of them had to stay in a double room while being induced. The story gets very complicated regarding the whys surrounding the births, but over the next three days, the two couples became very close friends sharing the one small room. The third couple was just down the hall. She delivered via Cesarean section the first night and had lots of company from the other four people coming in to visit her new baby. I felt like I lived at the hospital that week as I attended to my three couples.

*"There is power that comes to women when they give birth. They don't ask for it; it simply invades them. Accumulates like clouds on the horizon and passes through, carrying the child with it."*
**Sheryl Feldman**

## Shannon & Brian's Birth Story

Shannon and Brian were having their first baby and they hired me six weeks before the due date. It was important to them to have a birth plan.

*At her scheduled doctor's appointment the day before her due date, Shannon has an internal exam. Her cervix is thinned and the baby's head is still high. The doctor is concerned that the baby is going to be big. Shannon is fearful of whether she will be able to birth a big baby. There is no real, concrete evidence from the external exam that the baby is too big.*

*The doctor also mentions that if she has not delivered by next week, he would like to put gel on the cervix to ripen it, and the day after that he would like to induce labour.*

*It is five days after her due date: luckily no induction has occurred. Shannon starts to have mild contractions on her own in the morning. I explain she is probably in early labour; she could try walking. I suggest going to the mall and window shopping. This will help the contractions intensify and become closer and more regular. Shannon takes my advice. The mall is a great place to go in early labour; there are benches to sit on, lots of distractions and places to have a snack or a drink.*

*After the mall Shannon and Brian have a fairly quiet evening at home. Around midnight the mucus plug comes out and contractions start. They come approximately every four minutes; Shannon is shaking when having a contraction, but managing well.*

*I get the call to come to the house around 3:30 a.m. When I get there Shannon is a bit nauseated, but not throwing up. Nausea is typical during labour. It does not mean that a woman will throw up, but in the later stages of labour throwing up can be a good indication that mum is progressing and it usually helps to dilate the cervix. We start to count contractions to see how many she is having every ten minutes—they are four minutes apart.*

> *It is important to keep mum well-hydrated. If mum gets dehydrated she produces ketones in her urine and her body doesn't work as effectively. Care providers will want to give her an I.V. with saline solution. She can run the risk of having a high fever. Ideally we never want to see an I.V. They are uncomfortable on the arm or hand that they go in, and make movement more difficult especially at the pushing stage.*
>
> *I have included the recipe for "Labour Aid" in the back of the book. The mixture provides more than just plain water for a labouring mum. Some other options to give mum include Popsicles, frozen grapes, blueberries or other frozen fruit. It is typical that, once in active labour, a woman is not interested in eating.*

*To keep Shannon's energy up I make her some toast and have her drink watered-down juice. Her heartburn is worse so Brian gives her heartburn tablets which seem to help. Brian and I walk with Shannon, circling the inside of their home—up the hall, around the living room, thru the kitchen, all the while watching the news on the television repeat itself over and over. There is absolutely nothing to watch on television at 4:30 in the morning.*

*8:00 a.m.: Shannon gets a sharp pain in her belly and wonders if she should go to the hospital. We have been walking with short breaks for four hours. Concern is starting to show on her face, so we pack the car and head to the hospital.*

*There is no rush to get to the hospital. Sometimes I race to the hospital following dad's car and trying not to lose them. My fear is that dad will take a different turn and lose me and pull over to the side of the road and mum will deliver. This is not the case today.*

*Shannon has been labouring really well, but a change of venue is going to be good for her. The weather outside is wet and cold—it is early spring and walking outside is not an option.*

*Shannon is admitted and we are taken to our labour and delivery room. The car ride was a good distraction but she is still concerned about the size of her baby. We continue to walk the halls. She has not asked for any medication and is managing her contractions well.*

*It is 11:00 a.m. and the doctor finally comes in to check Shannon's cervix. To our delight she is 6-7 cm dilated and 90% to 95% effaced, meaning her cervix has almost completely thinned out. It is fabulous news that Shannon has progressed nicely.*

*At 1:30 p.m. Shannon is showing signs of hard work. Her contractions are three to four minutes apart and lasting a bit longer, so to provide some relief we decide to put her in the shower. She focuses on getting changed and into the shower.*

*Water is always a fabulous place for a labouring woman to be. Whether in a tub or shower, the warm water* cascading on a woman's stomach or back is extremely comforting. The second the water hits her belly it immediately reduces her discomfort. Shannon is still experiencing pain, but from what we can see on her face, she looks like she is feeling much better.

2:30 p.m.: Shannon gets out of the shower, and the doctor checks her progress. We are told she is 9 cm dilated, and her membranes are bulging. The doctor says if he can break the membranes it should speed up the dilation to 10 cm. The contractions will become stronger and quicker. Shannon agrees to the procedure.

At 2:50 p.m. the doctor uses something that looks like a knitting needle or a plastic chop stick with a rather small hook on the end. Neither mum nor baby feels anything. The poke to the membranes releases the waters, which were in the way of the baby's head. The fluid is clear, and mum's contractions get much stronger immediately; she asks if she can have something for the increased intensity.

Shannon is offered nitrous oxide—"laughing gas," similar to what a dentist would give his patients, but in a different concentration. The effect for women in labour is that it takes the edge off of the contraction. The bonus is that after a deep cleansing breath of fresh air, it is gone from a mum's system.

In another position change at 4:10 p.m., we put mum on the toilet. This gives her a chance to relieve herself and make more room in the pelvis for baby to move closer. This position is usually ideal for women; it is easier to sit upright and have her legs apart—all good for helping baby descend.

At 4:40 p.m. Shannon wants to return to the bed.

5:00 p.m.: After getting her in bed the doctor checks one more time. Mum is 10 cm dilated and ready to start pushing.

*Shannon is lying on her side and we turn her from side to side several times after a couple of contractions on each side. We guide her on how to hold her breath. She has not had medication, the gas has been put away and Shannon has to hold her breath through this stage of labour.*

*A woman's natural response about when to push kicks in and she works with her body to help the baby to descend and come through the pelvis.*

*At 5:54 p.m. an 8 lb 7 oz baby girl, Kaitlyn, is born. Shannon only pushes her first baby for 54 minutes. Kaitlyn is checked by the nurses. All her vital signs are perfect and she is returned to mum, skin-to-skin. Breast-feeding is instinctual for babies; they "smell" or sense their way onto the breast and to the nipple.*

*It is a fairly quick first birth. Afterwards we talk about how Kaitlyn's head is not as big as the doctor anticipated. It is so unfortunate that Shannon had to worry about this comment for the last week of her pregnancy.*

## Two Years and Three Months Later

I am hired again! I love being rehired and I loved Shannon and Brian's first labour. There are other considerations when a sibling comes along. Firstly, who is going to look after the first child at home when mum and dad race to the hospital? "Race" is a good term to use because second and third babies come faster and easier.

It seems that women can manage through their labour contractions more effectively, partly because the fear factor has gone, and they know they can handle the labour and delivery.

*Kaitlyn's grandma flies in from across the country twelve days before the due date, just in case she is needed early. Grandma also likes the idea that she gets quality time with Kaitlyn before the new baby is born. The scenario is especially fortunate for Shannon and Brian as they don't have to concern themselves with what to do with Kaitlyn if they need to leave in the middle of the night.*

*I visit with Shannon to discuss the birth. Shannon advises me that the baby is head down, and this is great. Sometimes when baby is breech, or bottom down, we try to give mum suggestions on how to get baby to turn. This baby has been head down for several weeks, but keeps changing from OA to OP.*

---

*Occiput Anterior (OA) is when baby's spine is facing front—the ideal position. In the Occiput Posterior (OP) position, baby's spine is lying directly on mum's spine, which will cause back labour. If the baby is OP, I have mum rocking on her hands and knees daily to help baby get into the OA position and nicely placed in the pelvis in anticipation of birth.*

*Doulas, with help from other practitioners, have a whole lot of tricks to help mum move baby out of the breech, or bottom down position. I mention this later in the book.*

*There are a handful of doctors in my area that are more open to a woman labouring and attempting a breech delivery. It used to mean an automatic Cesarean section every time, and at most hospitals it still does. The choice for women to try a breech delivery can be very satisfying even though it is a harder labour. Women weigh the odds of that against having a Caesarean section, which is a major surgery delivery.*

---

*Mum and I are having tea and reminiscing about the first labour. She mentions that when she walked into the hospital for Kaitlyn's birth, she tensed up. She felt like it made her stall getting to full dilation. I was curious about that as I didn't think she really had a problem with dilation slowing down. Shannon's labour was 18 hours from when she lost her plug until Kaitlyn's birth—not a time frame I would consider a long birth.*

*There is no correlation between losing the mucus plug and when labour starts. The mucus plug can dislodge itself two weeks before or an hour before labour; it is just an indication that your body is getting ready.*

*My confusion about the stall is answered when she explains that she believed it would hurt more when she was going to push and so was hesitant and tried to hold off. Also when we did the traditional three breaths per contraction, then holding each breath and pushing, she couldn't find her rhythm. (Her suggestion to me was that she only needed to take two breaths for each contraction and when it came time for this second delivery it worked extremely well.)*

*Three days before her due date, at her weekly appointment, the doctor does an internal exam and Shannon is already 3 cm dilated. I get a call at 9:30 a.m. the next morning. Shannon has been having mild contractions every 15 minutes lasting only 10 seconds – nothing to worry about yet – and she is feeling some back pain. There is also some bloody show and mucus, but she feels like she can "wait until tomorrow when her doctor will be on call." I love when clients tell me things like that; it says she is perfectly content and not at all worried that labour is on its way. A confident women preparing for birth!*

*I call a couple of hours later to see how things are progressing. Shannon tells me that there is only slight change in the contractions: they are now 20 seconds long, but still 15 minutes apart.*

*5:45 p.m.: I get a phone call telling me that things have changed: Can I please come to the house? I am ready to go and it is rush hour so I immediately get in my car and leave. Twenty minutes into my drive I get a call saying, "things have changed, and contractions have picked up," so they are going directly to the hospital.*

*I meet Shannon and Brian at the hospital. She can hardly walk, so we take her directly to the elevator and straight up to labour and delivery. After leaving them in the room, I run back downstairs to give the hospital Shannon's admission information. I finish and run back upstairs. The nurse has been trying to get an I.V. into Shannon's hand and is not doing very well. Shannon is in full-blown labour.*

*Thankfully the nurse leaves the I.V. to go get the on-call doctor. Brian and I take Shannon to the toilet. She feels like she needs to be there. The doctor walks in and we help get Shannon back to the bed for an assessment. The doctor advises us that mum is 10 cm dilated and ready to push.*

*Within eight minutes of being assessed, a beautiful baby girl is born at 7:18 p.m. Water breaks just moments before baby's head crowns; this time mum pushes two times and then breathes Brooke out. Brooke has a very short cord and as dad cuts it, mum lets out a huge sigh of relief. Mum has been holding her baby suspended above her tummy. We put baby straight to mum's chest, skin-to-skin. Brooke breast-feeds on both sides, each for half an hour.*

*Two hours after the birth Shannon gets up out of bed, showers and puts on a fresh gown. We sit mum in a wheelchair, to follow protocol, and wheel her down to the same private postpartum room she stayed in with Kaitlyn.*

*When I go to do my postpartum visit, we talk about the birth. Shannon comments that she should have told Brian to get her to the hospital when her contractions changed at 4:00 p.m., but she wanted him to finish his dinner first.*

*Then as Brian drove in rush hour traffic like Mario Andretti, he was reassuring mum that she wouldn't have the baby in the car, because "her water had to break first." The comforting words seemed to work for Shannon. I'm not sure she understood what he was saying, but he gave her a plausible excuse.*

This is why I am a doula—people living and enduring through times like this, and keeping focused, thoughtful and caring. I see loving couples daily. We are all stressed at times, but how people step up to the plate and shine amazes me. I look up toward the clouds and thank the Universe for such blessings and miracles.

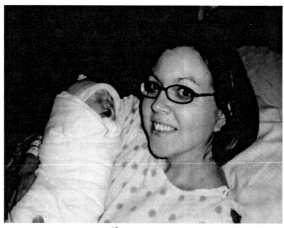

Shannon

# 3. Doula Information

*"I discovered I always have choices and
sometimes it's only a choice of attitude."*
**Judith M. Knowlton**

IT'S A CHALLENGE WHEN A WOMAN is not aware of her needs during labour – so how does she go about taking care of them? When a woman reads about the impending birth of her baby, doubt and worry can enter her thoughts. She may wonder whether she has been healthy enough during pregnancy, or if she has been eating and exercising enough, and doing all the other prescribed things she is told to do.

Books with positive pointers and advice like this one (together with my birth journal for your thoughts on the pregnancy) are two great ways to prepare for birth. Information is easily accessible through the Internet and should be used to research some of the medical facts. Care providers should be readily available to answer questions in a way that best suits the individual family.

I talk to women and find out why there might be concerns about the impending birth. I try to dispel any worries and explain that although the day will be long and hard the prize at the end, a gorgeous baby, is more than worth the effort. Engaging the services of a doula to guide and encourage mums-to-be and their husbands through the labour process makes it all much easier.

A well-trained doula who has attended a lot of births will be equipped to handle most situations that can arise; for example, what to do with posterior positioning of the baby or when to make position changes for mum. Preparing ahead of time for labour is an invaluable exercise.

Guidance with informative books, DVDs, CDs and charts all contribute to women's knowledge about the process of labour and delivery, empowering them to be more comfortable. In addition to prenatal classes, everything extra helps, and doulas can offer this to mum in prenatal visits.

## What a Doula Can and *Can't* Do

Most doulas here abide by a Code of Ethics and Standard of Practice set out by DONA International. The Code of Ethics ensures that the highest standard of integrity is maintained with clients as well as associates. This means respecting clients' privacy while working in their best interests, and maintaining professional respect for our colleagues.

In accordance with the Standard of Practice, doulas accompany women in labour to offer emotional, physical and informational support in all possible ways. Doulas act as advocates during labour and will advise, by referral, on matters such as breast-feeding and other clinical issues. Their professional development is ongoing so that they remain knowledgeable and up to date with industry changes.

During labour, doulas will have a lot of different techniques they can perform depending on the immediate needs. See the list in *Services a Doula May Offer* further along in this chapter, and please note this is only a short list. Each doula has a full list of individual specialties and techniques, and this is something to ask about during the initial interview.

A doula will *not* perform any clinical or medical tasks such as vaginal cervical checks or blood pressure checks, nor will she offer medical advice. Care providers should always be consulted. A doula will not take the place of mum's partner, but will strive to help partners participate more fully at the birth, according to personal comfort levels.

> *"If I had my life to live over, instead of wishing away nine months of pregnancy, I'd have cherished every moment and realized that the wonderment growing inside me was the only chance in life to assist God in a miracle."*
> **Irma Bombeck**

## Seeing a Change

When I walk into a labour and delivery room for the first time, I often see a woman who is not managing her contractions well suddenly stop, look at me and change. When she sees me enter she immediately relaxes and her stress level decreases. Then with a heavy sigh she says, "Thank you for coming" or "I'm so glad you're here." Her breathing slows and she waits for me to give her direction. I love that I can make a difference, but I also understand that this is the time for dad and I to get busy and help ease mum's discomfort. After a few questions dad and I plan how we will get mum to relax and slide into a nice groove of breathing with her contractions.

I have also witnessed position changes in the pushing stages of labour. Constant gentle reminders to breathe and relax can make an enormous difference for a woman during labour. I am often told that the sound of my voice was all she needed to hear to get her through that last hardest part. Sometimes a woman stares into my eyes as she is pushing, and I see the fear fade away.

You may be wondering where dad is—good question! He is most likely standing right beside mum and holding her hand. Whatever a woman fixates on in labour is acceptable, and never has a dad felt that I was taking over his place. Dad is always actively participating and sometimes he even gets to enjoy watching the changes his wife's body is going through while she is pushing. Dads get to watch the birth while I stay at mum's head and encourage her to push.

Doulas empower pregnant women, allowing them to understand the process and be more comfortable with what is happening to their bodies before, during and after giving birth.

## Doula Certification

There are lots of doula training bodies that offer certification. The most significant part for new doulas is the practical training received each time they enter into a labour and delivery experience. This remains the best part of the job. Something new will be learned every time. The elements experienced by each mum and baby in each birthing event are forever unique. When your doula has been trained by a known institute, it will indicate that she has achieved a high level of training and professionalism.

Doula training in British Columbia is done mainly at Douglas College, together with postpartum doula and breast-feeding training. Training is modeled after the Doulas of North America (DONA) Program. They offer training for doula certification for both birth and postpartum doulas. Visit DONA online at *www.dona.org*.

ALACE, Association of Labour Assistants and Childbirth Educators, offers training workshops and certification programs for Labour Assistants and Childbirth Educators. Learn more at *www.alace.org*. Their training is being offered by IBWP, The International Birth and Wellness Project.

Birth Works International (*www.birthworks.org*) offers training for childbirth educators and doula certification.

Childbirth International offers training for Birth and postpartum doulas, childbirth educators and breast-feeding Counsellors. Find the group online at *www.childbirthinternational.com*.

I mention only a few with no personal agenda. There are many wonderful organizations that train; you only need to look online for a list of what is in your area.

In the summer of 2010 DONA awarded the South Community Birth Program:

> **The Annie Kennedy Award**
>
> *This DONA International Award recognizes excellence in a doula group. The recipient group has shown the unwavering vision necessary for a group of doulas to become and remain successful, to grow and to serve its membership. This group develops collegial relationships and works as a team to provide services within its community to benefit doulas and families. This group has established a model that can be recreated successfully by other groups. (Doula Group Award)*

*"When I was born I was so surprised*
*I didn't talk for a year and a half."*
**Gracie Allen**

# Hiring a Doula

What should you know about hiring your doula prior to interviewing? Begin by searching the Internet to find a list of doulas in your area. There may be contact information for an association branch and most, though not all, doulas have websites. An excellent resource in Canada and the United States is *www.doulamatch.net*. This website is user-friendly and gives lots of detail about doulas and their availability. All training organizations should list certified doulas in your city and/or country.

Some doulas periodically have a Doula Dating Night or get together. On these occasions, you can come to meet the doulas personally. Use this time to interview all those you feel you could be comfortable with as your doula. They also have brochures that contain information about themselves. This is an excellent opportunity to sit down for a brief period with each one and ask questions.

If you don't have Internet access, you could consult doctors and midwifery clinics, breast-feeding and postpartum clinics, prenatal classes, community centers, hospitals, books and libraries. Word-of-mouth information is also always helpful when starting your search.

Read the individual doula websites and make a detailed list of what is most important for you and your birth. Note what services are offered and the groups that individual doulas are associated with. Personalize your list to reflect your own needs. Then list the most interesting doulas you would like to interview by telephone. The initial call is the time to make sure you have your main questions answered.

The next step is to shortlist three or four doulas and set up face-to-face interviews with them. This meeting is part of the service and there should be no obligation to hire. A personal meeting is primarily about whether you are comfortable with a prospective candidate.

Think about the qualities that are most important to you, about how you would like your birth to be and be specific. Some things to ask your prospective doulas are:

- Where did the doula train and what type of certification does she have?
- What is the fee and what does that include?
- How many births has she attended?
- Is she available on your due date?

- If you are due in the summer or at Christmas time, make sure she is available. Like people in all professions, doulas schedule time off to be with their families.

- How many clients does she take at once? The realities surrounding birth are important to understand. For instance, I may have two clients with the same due date and one will deliver early while the other is late. Or, I can have a due date for the 10th and one on the 20th of any given month, but both might give birth one day apart or even the same day.

- Does she have a back-up doula, and can you meet her? All doulas should have a back-up in case of unexpected personal or family illness, or in case she is busy with another client. Your doula should offer an opportunity to meet her back-up or at least explain who the other doula is.

- Will she attend your birth at the hospital or in your home? Most doulas attend at both locations, but check to ensure she does.

- Does she have children, and will finding a babysitter be an issue for her? If babysitting is an issue for her you need to know about this and decide if it is acceptable. Most doulas with children co-ordinate back-up arrangements.

- Does she have a part-time job? This may make a difference in whether she can attend right away or have to use a back-up.

- What is her philosophy on birthing?

- How will she include your husband/partner and what will she do for him or her?

- Does she offer private prenatal classes? If so, how many classes, what does she cover and what will the cost be?

- Does she offer prenatal and postpartum visits, and how many?

- Does she write a birth story?

- Does she help with breast-feeding at birth? What kind of training does she have?

- Will she respect your wishes if you choose not to breast-feed?

- Will she support your birth wishes, such as having a water birth, observing religious practices or rituals, or choosing pain medication during labour? Be sure to ask about specific scenarios, such as trying the nitrous oxide, but staying away from epidurals.

- How can the doula help you stay mobile during your labour?

- Will she be able to be quiet or talk you through your labour, and will she be aware enough to know which of these is best for you in the moment?

- Does she offer postpartum work, or is she able to offer a postpartum doula referral?

During the initial telephone interview ask about fees, services provided and philosophy. The personal interview should occur with your partner present to interview the doula. Set up the interview either at your home if you are comfortable with that, or meet at a coffee shop that is mutually convenient.

The interview can last from 15 minutes up to an hour, but ensure that both you and your partner enjoy being with this woman. She should be a pleasure to talk to and someone you are comfortable with. The conversation during the live interview should flow easily and remembering to ask every single question shouldn't matter too much. If necessary, she can always be contacted with more questions after the decision to hire her.

More important than the content of the questions is making sure you feel a connection. The doula you hire will be guiding you through a very personal journey so follow your instinct until it says, "She will be the perfect person for us."

## Dads and the Doula

Dads almost always wonder if a doula will subtract from his involvement and leave him in the corner not allowing him to participate. We are actually becoming more popular, thanks to dads who know the answer to this question. They are helping to spread the word about us. They feel great having us there and they can be more confident in attending to their wives because we have allowed them to fully participate in her care.

There are times I find out that dad has brought his own set of issues, such as fear of needles, or he might faint at the sight of blood. Sometimes it is hard being confined to a hospital room for prolonged periods. During a long labour dad may want to take a nap. No matter what happens dads know they can have a break while their wife is labouring with a trusted woman committed to her comfort and care. Dad can slip out for that much-needed time away.

It's important for the mum to know that her husband is taken care of. The doula will make sure that dad takes a nap, eats, has bathroom breaks, makes a phone call or just gets a bit of fresh air. mum can relax and concentrate on her labour, creating a more comfortable scenario for the birthing couple. Anxiety is attached to the smallest details and mums don't need any of it.

Dads should be aware that a doula will help take the fear of the unknown out of labour. She will be encouraging while instructing dad on what to do and where it should be done. If mum needs massaging, the doula will show dad where and how strong the massage should be. A woman in labour can tolerate both a stronger, firmer massage on some specific parts of her body, and a gentle touch on other areas. A doula can help with the mysteries of both. In addition, she will have dad helping in ways he never would have known about. At times I just look at dad and tell him that the labour is perfectly normal and that mum is doing exactly what she should be doing. Hearing this confirmation is hugely reassuring and decreases dad's anxiety level.

If a long, complicated labour ends in a Cesarean section, having a doula come into the operating room is beneficial. The doula sometimes cannot come in, but the care provider can ask for her to be included. With dad's anxiety level heightened, I calm him by guiding him with instructions on what to do. I start by helping him with information about changing into scrubs, after which I'll sit with him and explain what is going to happen when we go into the operating room. When we are in the operating room I advise him about mum and the procedure. When he is asked to come and see the baby at the bassinette with the paediatrician, I can stay with mum, hold her hand, stroke her hair, and talk softly to her about her baby.

Minutes after the birth, I am available to take pictures of the new family. I accompany mum to the recovery room while talking about the procedure, and I help the nurse get mum settled. When mum and baby are ready, I'm there to help with getting breast-feeding started. I show dad how to hold the baby and do skin-to-skin with his new baby.

If a Cesarean section is necessary, consider asking the care provider to have the doula attend in the operating room so she can be there for you. Doulas know that each birth with the same couple is different. There are subtle changes, and we make a difference each time.

> *"You were obviously a huge help to my wife,*
> *but you were a huge help to me – we were in*
> *the assessment room for so long I would have*
> *gotten anxious if you weren't there."*
> **Simon (a grateful dad)**

## The Doula Fee

Many people wonder why doulas charge what they do. I suggest they think about the day of their wedding – the cost of the dress alone for this one-day event – then the price of the baby's new stroller or crib. These are expenses most couples don't think about because they are necessary in the event. You will always remember your baby's birthday; it's *the* most important day of your life! To have peace of mind with the right doula and knowing that her professionalism brings you a more informed and controlled labour is priceless. I will explain the rationale for the fee structure.

In my area, new doulas will often offer free services to acquire experience. New doulas offering free services will do this only for a short time as the job is extremely time-consuming and there are many expenses. The most common doula fees range between $300 and $1400 at the time of writing. Some doulas work part-time to supplement their income; however, there are lots of full-time doulas. When a full-time doula is charging a slightly higher fee, be assured she is worth the amount as this is her profession.

Some doulas require a contract for services, which will outline what she offers together with the payment schedule. I personally have never used one, but it is entirely up to the individual doula hired.

The time required per birth averages this way:

The initial telephone call or email, the interview, the hire, prenatal visits, the birth, postpartum visits, follow-up email and telephone conversations leading to the birth can average 50 hours. A multip will often require less time, providing it is not a VBAC. Doulas take emails and telephone calls whenever clients may need guidance and information, and we are on call 24/7, two weeks before and two weeks after the due date.

A professional doula pays for all her own expenses including instalments to her pension plan and income tax.

The skill and knowledge a professional doula provides, including the personal care involved in working toward a shorter birth with fewer drugs, is invaluable. Of course, there are unforeseen emergencies such as Cesarean sections, and they only add to the time a doula will be with her client, seeing her through.

Some may wonder why doulas love their work. Personally speaking, I know we are passionate about our role and often call ourselves "birth junkies." I love what I do and feel privileged to attend the birth of a new baby. I see and feel the joy of parents when they can put a face to a tiny being that grew from a moment of passion between two people and now, at long last, this perfect being is theirs to love unconditionally and forever.

So, yes, I quite happily jump out of bed at 3:30 a.m. and will drive down a cold, frosty road to attend a birth. I am grateful for, and love the fact that I never do the same thing twice. Every birth is different. I have no doubt because I witness this daily.

> *"My husband is my left hand*
> *and my doula is my right."*
> **from *Doulas Make a Difference***

# Services a Doula May Offer

Doulas come from a variety of backgrounds. Some I know are from other countries and have been doctors, nurses and midwives. Sometimes a doula's passion takes her into different healing modalities; it doesn't really matter how she has become a doula. The fact that you can access so many amazing talents from these women is to your advantage on achieving a beautiful natural birth.

Doulas offer a huge variety of services. They don't all offer everything, but below are some of the general talents a doula may have. Restricted space doesn't allow for great detail about each of these skills. Asking a doula about her specific style or technique will result in the best definitions of each skill.

- Visualization: this encompasses a huge variety of techniques. Ask the doula if and how she uses this in her practice. Start now by visualizing your perfect birth. Attach sticky notes all over the house, each one having a different positive saying, e.g., "I can easily birth my baby" and so on.

- Reflexology: how does this help and what is her technique?

- Breast-feeding counsellor: where did she train?

- Private prenatal classes: what type of classes are offered (Lamaze, Birthing from Within, etc.)? How much will they cost and what is covered?

- Relaxation techniques: where did she train and what does she offer?

- Infant massage: this is specialised so do ask about its benefits for the baby.
- Support/preparation classes for siblings before baby's arrival: does she offer this service or can she recommend someone who does?
- Support for watching siblings while you are in labour: traditionally, this is not part of a doula's role, but you can always ask.
- Acupressure: where did she train and how does this help?
- Acupuncture: where did she train and how does this help?
- Photography: still shots and video can be arranged, though, if your doula is involved with the birth she may not be readily available for video, but she should be able to take a few pictures.
- Placenta preservation: doulas will make sure that your placenta is preserved for you to take home. Ideas for your placenta could include making art or planting it in your yard or garden.
- Placenta encapsulation: can be dried and put into capsules. If your doula doesn't actually preserve she will know someone who can do this for you.
- Homeopathy: where did she train and how does this help?
- Mother blessing celebration: an event similar to a baby shower that brings family and friends of

the mum together to honour her passage into motherhood.

- Music: the style is personal preference and should be brought in by the couple, but sometimes the doula will have CDs in her bag.
- Books, CDs and DVDs: all reference material can be on labour and birth for you and/or your baby.
- Belly casting: before birth you can do a belly casting (and even decorate the plaster cast). This can be very beautiful and later displayed in your home.
- Henna decoration: of the tummy and hands (and other parts of your body as you choose).
- Prenatal or postpartum massage: there is a huge variety of different techniques – what does she offer and where did she take her training?
- Postpartum doula services: there are doula agencies that offer postpartum work exclusively. A birth doula with too many clients may be unable to include postpartum service but, if necessary, she will know who to refer you to.
- Baby sign language: very specialised – the doula may also be able to refer you to a class or reference material.
- Birth pool rentals: a doula may know where to rent a pool for a home birth.
- Different language-speaking doulas: this will be specified on respective websites, but ask for what you need.

# Tools of the Trade

A doula supports her clients fully during labour and into the first hour or two after birth. There are various tools a doula has in her doula bag to assist in labour. These are the more hands-on, smaller items that could be used:

- Massage tools
- Massage oils or creams (unscented)
- Robozo – like a big woven shawl that helps with repositioning the baby if he or she is posterior
- Music CDs
- Notepad and pen for keeping notes to help in writing a birth story
- Birth ball
- Hot water bottle or rice bag for heat therapy
- Hair ties, lip balm, mints and gum
- Flashlight
- Snacks, sometimes to be shared with dad

# Techniques

Each doula may choose to use certain techniques in her practice, and the choices are unique to each doula's expertise, training and ability. Here is a quick list of the more important things offered; after all, a doula doesn't only remind her clients to drink lots of fluids.

- Guidance for moving: in early labour a woman may be encouraged to stroll through the halls, or walk up and down stairs. This could also involve changing positions in the tub or shower, on the ball, on the bed, or standing.

- Helping both parents understand the when and why of what is going on from moment to moment. Also helpful are explanations about changes in mum and her body.

- Advice about when touch and massage are needed and how to apply them using hands or massage tools. I use massage so frequently that when a woman tells me how wonderful the foot massage was, I have to remember that I gave her one. I usually encourage dad to massage before I do; I feel it is more effective that way, but, more importantly it gives him the chance to care for mum.

- Advocacy of couple's wishes during labour and delivery.

- Specialised labour support with a posterior baby: to help the baby move into a more desirable position, I use a robozo, which is a specially woven long and wide scarf that fits gently over the belly. There are lots of different ways to move a baby from lying on mum's back to lying forward. In most cases, this technique will remove back labour discomfort.

- Acupressure on several different parts of the body: this can be good for melting cervical lips, enhancing contractions, aiding in the descent of the baby into the pelvis, fear and nausea, as well as helping to deliver the placenta. Specific training is needed.

- Acupuncture can be used with specific training and can be highly effective.

- Guidance about how and when to push: usually when you are at 10 cm dilated. This depending on how labour has progressed and there are numerous techniques.

- Breathing techniques for pushing: a woman might want to verbalize while her body does most of the work, or maybe she prefers to hold her breath and push.

- Position changes during the pushing stage: this is always good for helping the baby along and should be done every ten to fifteen minutes. It also helps to encourage mum when she doesn't want to move.

- Knowing when to advise slowing down to change breathing techniques. This is important especially when the baby (at 10 cm dilated) is coming too fast or with the urge to push prior to being examined to confirm 10 cm readiness.

- Counter pressure on the hips and back: this is beneficial to most women during different parts of her labour.

- Heat or cold as needed: this is about where and when to apply each—heat is more often used on the back and a cold cloth is used on the body, head and face.

- Help in the shower or tub: there is therapeutic value to having a woman take a shower or bath. Most people enjoy a spa, swimming, hot tub or pool, even a tub at home for relaxation. The same principle applies, in fact is intensified, for women in labour.

- Providing a safe, comfortable environment: a woman knowing she is in a safe place with people she trusts is invaluable. A doula will tactfully ask friends and family to leave or join the labour room as is comforting for the labouring woman.

- Aromatherapy: a doula must be specifically trained to offer this service. Please get the appropriate advice before you go into labour.

- Setting the mood with music: The doula will usually have something in her bag if the couple forgets to bring their own music. Most people bring computers, iPods and other musical devices into their births. At home, of course, anything goes.

- Controlling the lighting: even if the woman has not asked, the lighting can be dimmed to create a cosier environment for mum. Soft lighting is also a welcoming way for the baby to gently enter into the world. With home births, beeswax candles are best, but because of the nitrous oxide, they are not allowed at the hospital.

- TENS application: (transcutaneous electrical nerve stimulation): This involves a hand-held unit that the woman controls. Pads are applied to the back and electronic pulses help to distract and lesson the contractions. This is especially beneficial with back labour. Doula must have training.

These are only some of the services a doula can provide during labour. Because there are doulas with specialties in addition to birth coaching, research is the best way to find out what can be offered. Most will discover that doulas are truly talented women.

*"Just as a women's heart knows how and when to pump her lungs to inhale, and her hand to pull back from fire, so she knows when and how to give birth."*
**Virginia Di Orio**

## Postpartum Doulas

Some families prefer the aftercare offered by a postpartum doula, and there are plenty of certified women that can help. It doesn't matter if the baby was delivered via Cesarean section, mum needs extra help, or mum simply wants to enjoy some quality time with her baby without worrying about household chores and cooking. She may need breast-feeding help or guidance on setting up a nursery. Doulas can be available in the evenings to help with a fussy baby. Postpartum doulas are happy to help with all a woman's needs.

Postpartum doulas usually work in groups so they can offer round-the-clock service. The minimum is four hours and can continue to twenty-four-hour care. She may be hired for mum's care or baby's care. She can look after other children, perform light housecleaning tasks, cook, run errands or simply help to make the family's first few days or weeks a little easier.

Most have breast-feeding experience or training and can guide and educate a woman about everything she does for her baby. Doulas are there only to advise, encourage and support.

For information about postpartum doulas, ask the birth doula, care provider, prenatal instructor, hospital staff or friends, or simply go to *www.dona.org* to find Canadian and U.S. listings for postpartum doulas.

Pre-screen postpartum doulas over the phone first; then meet face-to-face with one or more. The interview should include the following points:

- The doula's education and training location.
- What overall services does she offer?
- Does she have references? Ask for names and numbers and make sure to call.
- The number of hours you require. If she can't accommodate, ask for a referral to someone who can make the time commitment.
- Is she available before and after your due date in case baby is early or late?
- What experience does she have?
- What are her fees? In my city postpartum doulas are charging between $20 and $30 per hour.
- If you know there will be a need, make sure she has specific breast-feeding training.

These women are well-trained and very talented and they have a broad range of services they can provide. They will change their routine to suit the woman, the baby and the family's changing needs throughout the time she is there. A birth doula can provide referrals and help with how to go about hiring a postpartum doula. When interviewing, the same principles apply: instincts will let you know the woman most personally suitable to come into your home to take care of you and your family.

One very important point to remember is that postpartum doulas do not help mum with clinical issues or postpartum depression. They are there for care and comfort and will help guide you to where you can get help, but it is most important that you see your care provider for medical attention.

> *"If I don't know my options, I don't have any."*
> **Diana Korte**

# The Sitting Month

Postpartum doulas are used in Canada because Canadians haven't quite yet grasped the advantage of engaging their families to help provide full-time care for mum and baby after birth. Within Asian culture, the first month home is called "the sitting month". It is seen as a period of confinement when mum stays home with her new baby and is looked after by her family. This care actually starts during labour. Before I get to my next birth story I would like to share the perfect article written by a woman named Hoai Do. She graciously has given me permission to include her article here, and I believe it will explain more fully the traditions that Asian women endeavour to keep during labour and when they go home.

I gratefully thank Hoai Do for allowing me to publish her article describing the sitting month:

"Women want to eat to get the energy before going through the labour. Western culture, however, discourages eating for fear a full stomach will induce nausea/vomit especially during active labour phase. This has been a common complaint for Chinese women. Many did not understand why they were not allowed to eat and thought the hospital policy is too strict. When asked for a drink of water, women were offered ice chips instead of warm water that they prefer. Most Chinese women will endure the thirst for fear the cold water from ice chip will upset their internal hot/cold balance and subsequently increase their risk of developing arthritis in old age.

Traditionally, men do not play a major role during deliveries. Husband/expectant fathers usually remain outside of labour room till the baby is born. Female family members/relatives such as mother, mother-in-law, aunts or sisters provide much of needed support during this time. This tradition is slowly evolving as extended family members/relatives are not readily available and nuclear families are becoming more prevalent. Younger and more Western acculturated couples will want to attend childbirth classes. Expectant fathers are more willing/wanting to stay in labour room with their wives to provide support and serve as labour coaches.

## Postpartum Practices

Chinese women believe strongly in postpartum practices. Caring for oneself immediately after childbirth is very crucial in restoring women's health to pre-pregnant condition. There are wide regimens of self-care and special food intake during postpartum period. A period of care right after the delivery ranging from one to three months is known as the "sitting month".

Depending on regional differences, there are variances in regiments and practices associated with sitting month. During the sitting month, women are to abstain from taking a bath, washing their hair, exposing themselves to cold water, cold temperature environment and wind, drinking ice water or eating "cold" food (i.e. uncooked vegetables, salads or fruits). The reasons for these restrictions are based on the beliefs that women are undergoing a cold stage right after the delivery due to loss of blood. In order to restore the energy, women need to consume food that are considered "hot" (i.e. hot water, soups, ginger, wine and food that are high in protein) and avoid exposing themselves to cold air, cold water or wind.

Western providers and health care members who are unfamiliar with sitting month have a difficult time in understanding the Chinese women who just gave birth. In Western culture, cold drinks such as milk, orange juices, ice water and cold food such as salad, cold sandwiches, tomato-based sauce dishes and desserts such as Jell-O, fruits and ice cream are routinely offered to women during their in-patient stay. In contrast, for Chinese women these are the types of food that their mothers, women friends and relatives have advised avoiding as much as possible. Women who had Cesarean section would want to avoid not only "cold" food but also beef or seafood. Beef and seafood are believed to prolong the healing process. It is not unusual for hospital staff to find the food served left untouched. In-patient women preferred to have their food brought in from home. For women who have an episiotomy, nurses will advise women to use ice packs to reduce swelling and inflammation. Young Chinese women who have been exposed to Western culture will heed the advice and adopt the practice. For the majority of Chinese women, however, the practice is considered contradictory to their Chinese health belief. Traditionally, women should avoid using anything cold for fear that cold compress will increase their risk of incontinence, headache, backache and/or arthritis in old age.

*Chinese Cultural Profile*, author(s): Hoai Do, MPH, Harborview Medical Center/University of Washington. Date authored: June 01, 2000, *www.ethnomed.org*

## Birth Story – Anonymous

*Mum is Korean and dad is Chinese – a nice, quiet couple who live with dad's mum. Mum is in good health, open to drugs, looking for a natural labour but is a bit nervous. Mum works in the health care system and knows the care providers are often overworked. She realizes having me as her doula will make a huge difference in her care, and her anxiety about a hospital birth lessens.*

*Mum starts early labour a day before her due date. She is having irregular contractions. She has been walking to help bring on established labour all day, alternating with sitting in the shower. By 7:30 p.m. I get the call to come over. Dad is concerned that mum has been labouring all day with contractions five minutes apart and is working hard. Dad thinks she is getting too tired and wonders if we need to go to hospital. I arrive at their home within the hour and am introduced to grandma, a lovely and obviously concerned woman. Grandma has been cooking all day and is waiting in anticipation to do more for our labouring mum.*

*I notice mum's contractions aren't too difficult but are consistent with early labour. At this point the best thing she can do is get some sleep, as impossible as it sounds. I tell her to contact the on-call care providers at the hospital; they will advise her about how to nap. I know the advice the care providers will give, but it is beyond my scope of practice to directly advise mum. I give emotional and physical support, leaving all medical advice to the care providers. I leave, telling them I will be available during the evening and that they can call if they need help.*

*I arrive at the hospital the next day at 3:30 p.m. Mum and dad are in the assessment room. The hospital is big and on this day it is busy. There are no nurses available upstairs where the newer rooms with the fabulous birthing tubs are located. So we do the "corridor walk," appropriately named by one of the doctors. I'm sure he suggests that walk to every labouring mum.*

*Back and forth, down all the numerous halls—not long, but we don't walk very fast. Trainloads of clean laundry pass us. Nurses and doctors buying coffee, and people coming to visit all walk by. But mum is oblivious to all. We stop every few minutes to comfort mum and I remind her to breathe.*

*At 4:30 p.m. our midwife finds us and tells us we have a room available now. We walk down another hall, and take the elevator back up. Mum has had enough walking and I start to fill the tub. She is exhausted but we've managed to get contractions closer together and stronger.*

*Mum stays in the tub for an hour and a half, laying on her back and sides. We turn her to her hands and knees and she suddenly has a huge and long contraction (the beauty of position changes)—we warm up the tub again.*

*At 6:30 p.m. she's had had enough of the tub for now and we get her out, moving her to a birthing ball. Then she asks for the nitrous oxide.*

*7:30 p.m.: Mum is checked for progress and is at 6 cm dilated. Her cervix is paper thin (totally effaced) and the midwife believes it would be best to rupture her membranes to get dilation progressing a bit faster.*

*8:30 p.m.: Mum goes back into the tub and this time the gas is handy. We give verbal support while mum is contracting and lying in the tub.*

*9:20 p.m.: Mum has had enough of the tub again and gets out. We put her back on the ball, sitting and leaning against the bed. (Keeping mums upright is always the best position. Walking at this point is usually not possible—she is just too tired to stand). Mum lasts only 20 minutes in this position before we move her to the toilet, which is typically difficult for mums at this stage, and then we put her into bed.*

*10:20 p.m.: Mum is checked; she is still at 6 cm and her cervix is starting to swell. The midwife believes that if mum has an epidural her body will have time to relax enough for the cervix to start to thin and dilate again.*

*11:00 p.m.: The anaesthesiologist, a doctor mum has worked with in the past (she is a nurse in this hospital) has arrived to give her the epidural. Mum feels comforted by the fact that she knows and respects the doctor and the epi is put in quickly. The doctor gives her a big hug and her congratulations before leaving.*

*12:20 a.m.: Mum is finally settled and comfortable. She eats a Popsicle while dad and I get ourselves comfortable preparing to have a nap in the room. We do this knowing that the nurse stays beside mum, monitoring her and doing her charting.*

*1:10 a.m.: The midwife returns to check on mum, but there is no progress. Oxytocin is ordered. We wait until 3:20 a.m. for the on-call obstetrician to come up. Mum is assessed again according to protocol, and before the Oxytocin can be administered*

*5:20 a.m.: Mum is checked again and is now at 7 to 8 cm dilated and +1. Oxytocin is continued.*

*The midwife is not a medical doctor so she cannot order the Oxytocin. The +1 measurement describes how low the baby's head is in the pelvis. The cervix dilates from zero to 10 cm. Effacement refers to the cervix thinning. It will be 100% effaced, which is paper thin. These two things must happen before a woman is totally dilated and can start to push.*

*At 7:10 a.m, Mum is now 9 cm dilated. Fabulous news!*

*8:05 a.m.: There is a shift change, so we get a different midwife and a second midwife who is doing her practicum.*

*8:15 a.m.: Grandma enters the room, bringing dad and I noodles for breakfast. I've never had this type of breakfast, and I find it heavenly. I share mine with one of the midwives; we're both hungry. Grandma comes over to me, knowing that I've been with her son and daughter-in-law all night. She proceeds to give me an amazing shoulder and neck rub. I am wishing she was my own grandma! Her actions are thoughtful and sweet. She has also brought special food and tea for mum to have after the birth.*

*Mum has been indicating for the last hour and a half that she is getting close to pushing, so the midwife slows down the epidural until the contractions are just manageable. The midwife wants mum to have a "walking epidural" to ensure that she will have feeling in her legs and so she can feel and sense the urge to push. This works effectively for our mum.*

*At 9:45 a.m. Mum is checked again and is now 10 cm dilated, and ready to push. We give her a small snack of ice cream and apple juice, both cold, but it is the only nourishment she takes willingly, knowing that the final stage of pushing is upon her.*

*10:35 a.m.: Mum starts to push. She is on her back with "labour links," a clever device designed to hold onto like a water ski rope on the birthing bar. The bar is placed on the bed to give mum a grip while lifting herself into an upright position to hold her breath and push deep into her bottom. We've tried her on her hands and knees, squatting, and then side lying.*

Finally, mum is tested to see if she can walk to the toilet. She passes the hospital protocol for a "walking epidural" and moves with guidance toward the washroom, which is just behind a small partition 10 feet from the bed.

Sitting on the toilet is an excellent position. Mum can be upright and her legs are wide apart so that she can sometimes even pee which makes just that much more room for the baby's head to slip down further into the pelvis.

We gather around mum to cheer her on and to comfort her. I stand beside her while she is seated and gently massage her shoulders and back. The midwife squats on the floor in front of her watching to see if there is any change in the perineal area. Dad, of course, is right there beside mum.

Suddenly, the midwife advises that we need to get mum back to the bed. Mum has only been sitting for about 15 minutes, but I hear the urgency in the midwife's voice. We abruptly get mum up and moving toward the bed.

The upright movement brings the baby's head down farther, and the midwife sees it crowning. Half way to the bed she starts to call out instructions. I guide mum, the nurse is calling for assistance on her phone, and the second midwife gathers and opens the proper tools on the tray for delivery.

The midwife looks at dad and asks, "Do you want to catch your baby?" A very startled dad, who all along has been a constant, confident and caring partner, confusedly answers, "Yes!" Immediately, the midwife thrusts his arms down beside mum's legs. She is now standing at the bed delivering the baby.

The bag of waters explodes onto the floor; what the midwife broke before was only the fore waters. The midwife is behind and dad is beside mum as they jointly catch the *baby. Dad is then instructed to hold his baby with both hands and we move to pick mum up and place her on the bed, all the while we watch not to get in the way of the cord.*

*The birth occurs at 1:17 p.m. and the placenta is delivered at 1:23 p.m. Dad, with the help of the midwife, places the baby onto mum. There are now more nurses in the room and they look at the perfect newborn baby on mum's chest. They begin to clean up the floor. Not many instruments had been needed and some of the equipment is being rolled outside the room.*

*I help mum begin breast-feeding her beautiful healthy daughter, as the midwife looks on to see if mum has torn or needs any medical attention with suturing.*

*The best part about this birth has been that even with the slower progress throughout the night, the care providers took an active approach by helping a tired mum's cervix have a break and for her to have a nap. When it came time to push she had been given the two-plus hours, lots of position changes, and the end result was an easy, very quick delivery.*

*Baby breast-feeds on both sides, and I make sure that mum and dad have eaten something. Sometimes mums get only a slice of toast and cup of tea in the middle of the night, but this couple has been treated well with grandma's cooking.*

*When all the care providers have finished and leave the room, I leave as well, always getting a hug and thank you from mum, who now says, "I couldn't have done this without you." Truly, this is the best compliment and puts a smile on my face, while knowing that it was indeed mum who did the work. Then I get a bigger hug from dad and he thanks me.*

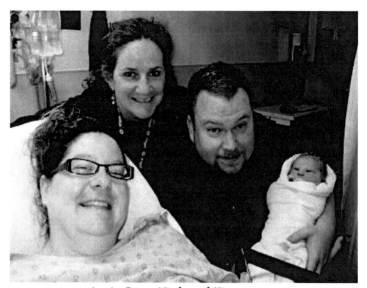

Angie, Ryan, Neala and Kim

# 4. Birth Plan or Preferences

*"The parallels between making love and giving birth are clear, not only in terms of passion and love, but also because we need essentially the same conditions for both experiences: privacy and safety."*
**Sarah Buckley**

NOT ALL MY CLIENTS WANT ONE, but I enjoy helping them put together a birth plan. I explain that birth takes on a life of its own and will easily divert itself, so not to rely heavily on the plan. It is nice to share with the care providers when you are in labour, and for your peace of mind.

I email my clients blank birth plans, showing different styles. There is a lot of information to choose from and to use to personalize the plan. My recommendation for the birth plan is point form, easy to read and only one page. The care providers prefer short and concise because they are very busy.

*"Don't forget to tell people that they shouldn't rely on their birth plan. Too much can happen and it has to be discarded."*
**A client's suggestion**

I encourage you to think about some of your options. I stress; ask when you are not clear on the procedures, for example, there are pros and cons to waiting for the umbilical cord to stop pulsing before it is cut. I ask you to do the research and ask for clarification from your care provider. Your doula can help with much of the birth plan but should be referring you when it is a clinical question. Some or most of these ideas may already be standard practise in your hospital.

## Birth Plan Sample

Your name ........................................................................

Husband/partner's name ............................................

Due date .........................................................................

Doctor or midwife's name ..........................................

Doula's name ................................................................

This is our first (second, third, etc. pregnancy)

Brief outline of your specific expectations:

❑ We want to experience a water birth

❑ We want a totally drug-free labour

❑ Both my husband / partner and doula will help guide me with position changes and other comfort measures during labour

❑ My husband / partner and my doula will be the only ones attending my birth, or (include other names of family & friends) might also be there

❑ Please keep us informed about the progress of labour

❑ I would like a mirror to watch my baby crowning

❑ I want freedom of movement; use the Doppler for monitoring every 15 minutes

❑ I don't want to be lying in bed strapped in for constant monitoring if there is no medical reason

❑ I don't want any medical students, interns, residents or non-essential personnel present during my labour or the birth

❑ We would like the room to be dimly lit; please turn all unnecessary lights off

❑ We would like soft music playing; I will be bringing my own

❑ If necessary, I would like to start with the nitrous oxide

❑ Pain medication – please don't give me anything for pain unless I ask – please tell me what my options are

❑ I prefer to try natural methods of pain relief first before being offered drugs

❑ My thoughts on episiotomy – a tear or a cut – are … (this is a very personal topic and you should talk to your care provider before labour about protocol and philosophy)

❑ Immediately after birth (provided there are no complications) I want skin-to-skin contact; please leave the baby to find the breast. Please wait to have baby weighed and measured

❑ I wish to delay (or skip) the application of eye ointment so my baby and I can have skin-to-skin contact (this may be optional in your area; ask your care provider why you would decline eye ointment)

❑ I wish to delay (or skip) the Vitamin K shot so my baby and I can have skin-to-skin contact (Vitamin K is optional and is available in liquid form—discuss it with your care provider)

❑ I would like to try using the following birth aides (ie; birthing ball, meditation, massage, aromatherapy, Reiki, music, visual aids, nipple stimulation, etc.)

- ❏ For my comfort I prefer to labour in the shower or tub for as long as possible
- ❏ I would like to wear my glasses at all times
- ❏ Please keep vaginal exams to a minimum unless needed
- ❏ I prefer not to have the membranes ruptured artificially unless it is necessary (ask your care provider about this)
- ❏ I would like a warm compress applied to the perineum to help ease the crowning of the baby
- ❏ I would like to wait until my body gives me the urge to push at 10 cm dilation
- ❏ I would like to breathe my baby out, with gentle pushes
- ❏ I would like to make grunting or other noises as my body may feel compelled to voluntarily do at the time of pushing
- ❏ My husband / partner would like to help catch our baby
- ❏ My husband / partner would like to cut the cord
- ❏ I would like to allow time for the cord to stop pulsing before being cut
- ❏ If I need a C-section or other medical treatment, dad will follow baby and spend time skin-to-skin with baby
- ❏ If I need a C-section I want my doula present with my husband / partner and I in the operating room
- ❏ If I need a C-section or there is another complication, please do / not give my baby a bottle / formula supplement. I prefer my baby receives expressed breast milk or my expressed colostrum
- ❏ I want to keep my placenta (you may want to plant this in your garden / make art work to display in your home / encapsulate for use later on)
- ❏ I want to keep baby with me at all times while in hospital

A birth plan has a purpose, although it is not always used or even considered in the moment. Sometimes mum just says, "Yes" to the impending Cesarean with a "Get this baby out now!" There is still validity in doing a birth plan for the women who want one.

## Going Into Labour

Going into labour and the birth process are natural bodily functions. When you get excited at a happy event like a sporting game and you jump up and down or hoot and holler, it's a natural response. When you are not feeling well, you might take something from the medicine cabinet after listening to what your body is telling you. Your body usually takes care of itself automatically and reacts on its own. The same process happens when you are having a baby.

I am frequently asked, "When will I go into labour?" Your body does it naturally. There are hundreds of subtle signs and some or all may apply to you, but you still may not know you are almost there until you actually go into labour. When this happens, first call your care provider and they will advise you. You can call your doula, and she will be able to answer easy questions. Often she can give you suggestions to help quicken the process of early labour. Listing every scenario about early labour is extensive. Just remember to call someone.

Allow your body to move through each stage of labour. Have trusting support, and be guided, as you slowly become more focused within.

*Breathe and Believe!*

# Breast-feeding

It's essential to have good breast-feeding education before the birth. Understanding about the latch is the most important part to breast-feeding. I wish prenatal classes spent more time on the subject, but understandably they have a lot to cover. Find a doula with breast-feeding training and ask her to include this in her prenatal visit. Ensure this component is part of your preparation for birth. Doulas with training will help you and baby achieve a good latch at birth, to prevent breast-feeding issues later on when you go home.

I show Dr. Jack Newman's DVD called *Visual Guide to Breastfeeding*, to all my clients. This particular DVD answers a lot of questions, uses good visuals and advises what to do if you have any concerns or complications. It is currently my favourite breast-feeding visual. Clients comment that this has definitely helped explain more about the process.

We review the content and I answer questions my clients have. It is important to understand what breast-feeding will look like before baby is born. The first few weeks at home are chaotic enough.

Le Leche League is another great resource. The Le Leche League outlines a great deal of information about breast-feeding, including fascinating aspects of the dynamics of the breast, information on breast pumps, storage of breast milk, positioning, fussy babies, multiple babies and breast-feeding, nipple and breast problems, and a whole lot more. The group has neighbourhood La Leche League group meetings regularly, where other new mums come to meet and talk about breast-feeding issues. Le Leche League Leaders are trained breast-feeding consultants. Primary care givers, hospitals, community centers, birth doulas and postpartum doulas are there to help. Websites can provide many answers to questions about breast-feeding: *www.drjacknewmann.com* or *www.llli.org*. Always look for advice sooner than later.

Most women can breast-feed. Sometimes women who have had breast augmentation or reduction surgery can experience problems that result from the reconstruction of the nipple, and that affect the milk ducts. Please discuss this with all care providers including lactation consultants before baby arrives so that you know all your options and are well taken care of.

Standard practise at BC Women's Hospital & Health Centre in Vancouver is that every uncomplicated vaginally birthed baby goes directly to mum's chest skin-to-skin. Babies are given the chance to acquaint themselves with their surroundings; they instinctually have a sense to suck. I have watched babies wiggle themselves to find the nipple and start suckling. Babies will stare at mum and can recognize her voice then move their head to look in the direction of dad's voice.

I will take pictures in the first half hour, capturing these precious moments while mum is first trying to breast-feed. If Cesarean section is necessary and the baby will not be with mum in recovery, please suggest dad go into the nursery and hold the baby skin to skin until mum is reunited with baby.

It's important to allow baby to start this sucking process, but it should be noted that babies are not hungry when they are born. Babies can go up to 24 hours in some cases without going to the breast to eat. It's an instinctual need to suck right after birth, which in turn helps to start mum's milk production.

A baby needs this good start to his or her life. The colostrum, "the first milk", is concentrated, thick, sticky and golden in colour. It has a high concentration of nutrients and immunities and the small amount immediately available is the perfect quantity for baby's tiny chick-pea-sized tummy. As the stomach grows so does milk production—Mother Nature at her best!

A common question from clients is, "Is baby getting enough?" At birth, yes, of course he is. Putting baby to the breast often, for as long as baby is interested, will help to start milk production. It will take about three days for your milk to come in. By then your baby's tummy has expanded and can handle the higher volume. If baby is losing weight it could be for a variety of reasons. It is important to contact your care providers to help you find out why.

Colostrum acts as a natural laxative. It helps to rid the baby's system of the black tar-looking bowel movements, called meconium. If this is not cleansed from the body quick enough the baby could become a bit jaundiced, meaning that his bilirubin counts are high. The doctor may recommend putting baby under a special sun lamp to clear up, meaning another possible day in hospital.

La Leche League International describes bilirubin as:

*More than half of all newborns become jaundiced within the first week of life, which is why this jaundice is called "physiologic", meaning normal. Physiologic jaundice is caused by a rise in blood levels of bilirubin, a yellow pigment that is a product of the breakdown of hemoglobin from the extra red blood cells with which most babies are born. Jaundice results when excess bilirubin accumulates in the blood and is deposited in the skin, muscles, and mucous membranes of the body, causing the skin to take on a yellowish colour.*

*Normal newborn (or physiologic) jaundice is caused by a combination of three factors: the increased amount of bilirubin produced in the newborn, the increased reabsorption of bilirubin from the intestines, and the limited ability of the newborn's immature liver to process large amounts of bilirubin as effectively as a more mature liver. The newborn's liver commonly takes a week or two to mature sufficiently to handle the build-up of bilirubin in the blood.*

*As the baby feeds well, feeds often (ten to twelve times per twenty four hours), passes stools, and the baby's liver processes the backlog of bilirubin in the baby's system, physiologic jaundice will gradually resolve on its own within several days or weeks. Physiologic jaundice is not a disease; it is a harmless condition that has no after effects, provided the baby's bilirubin does not reach unsafe levels.*

# Benefits of Breast-feeding

The Breastfeeding Committee for Canada lists several benefits of breast-feeding, including but not limited to the following:

- Mother's breast milk is made especially for her baby; formula can not compare.

- Baby's gut digests it easier, and causes fewer tummy problems.

- Economics: breast-feeding exclusively is free. There is no cost for formula or bottles, and no time spent washing and preparing equipment.

- The bonding time between mum and baby for feedings is irreplaceable. If, however, bottle-feeding is the way you will be feeding baby, try and feed baby skin-to-skin and as close to the breast as possible to get that natural feeling and bonding.

- Breast-feeding is a biologically efficient system providing nutritional, immunological and emotional nurturing for normal growth and development during the first years.

- Unique nutrients, enzymes, growth factors, hormones and immunological and anti-inflammatory properties of breast milk decrease the incidence/severity of respiratory disease, gastroenteritis, bacterial meningitis, urinary tract infections, botulism and low iron stores and anemia.

- Breastfeeding has a possible protective effect on Sudden Infant Death Syndrome, Crohn's Disease, ulcerative colitis, insulin dependent diabetes, lymphoma and allergic disease.
- Beyond infancy the ongoing benefits contribute to protection against obesity and to improved cognitive development.
- Breastfeeding reduces mum's risk of breast, ovarian and endometrial cancer, osteoporosis and anemia.

For a full list of benefits please look further into medical books and websites that go into greater detail.

I am passionate about breast-feeding. I understand that there are times it is not a choice for mum and formula feeding is essential. Have your care provider go over all the options; ask for help in the pharmacy or with a lactation consultant about bottles and formula.

When I was working at a grocery store I had a customer who knew I was a doula and breast-feeding consultant. She asked why her daughter was having so many problems with her baby's upset tummy. I noticed that the formula she was buying was supplemented with extra A+ iron. I suggested that she switch to regular formula of the same brand. A few days later I saw the customer again and she said her daughter was happy and baby had no more tummy problems. So when you think you are doing your baby a favor by buying the extra stuff included in a formula, it may be the cause of your baby's discomfort, and not necessarily the brand. Switch up until you get the correct one for baby.

## Breast-feed Comfortably

First and foremost mum needs a convenient place where she can sit upright with a straight back and her feet on the floor. More importantly, baby should be positioned close to the breast, at tummy/breast height and lying on a nursing cushion or pillows. Mum will suffer from fatigued, sore muscles if she has to strain to feed baby. This preparation is significant and should stay set up for mum for the first few weeks while she and baby become pros at feeding times. (The same goes for a bottle-fed baby.)

Mum should have a supply of all that she might want beside her within easy reach for feedings. Things like a water bottle and snacks like granola bars, nuts or fruit – anything non-perishable that can be left out – are important. It is also important for mum to keep her strength up; breast-feeding can take a lot out of her.

A telephone should be close by unless mum is comfortable not answering it when she is breast-feeding. She may want the remote controls for the television or music, or a book, and of course, easy access to light switches.

Ideally dad or someone else is at home and available to supply her with water or juice and light meals or snack food while she goes through the process of feeding baby. This will save her time and is most convenient.

The actual *how to* breast-feed your baby I will leave for the face-to-face care providers, doulas and prenatal educators. You need more than a paragraph to explain this process. Remember if you are not comfortable or are disappointed with one feeding, you will get another chance in a couple of hours. Please ask for help.

If you are experiencing tenderness on your nipples, you can buy cream specific to helping them stay moist and heal. There is always the quick and easy trick of expressing colostrum or milk and rubbing on the nipple, allow it to dry near the heat of a lamp or with a warm cloth. Take good care of the nipples, and if you have any problems get help quickly. They can chap and crack and breast-feeding at that point is said to be worse than labour.

When your milk comes in you may find that your breasts become overly full and engorged. Engorgement happens when the milk comes in quickly approximately two to three days after birth. You can help by putting frozen or cold green cabbage leaves, (red cabbage will stain you and your clothes) on the breast between you and your bra to help reduce the swelling. Also applying warm water in the shower or a warm cloth over the sink and expressing some milk can relieve the pressure. You might consider expressing and storing the extra milk.

This part of the milk production process doesn't last long, so get proactive right away. Otherwise you may develop mastitis: an illness that can become severe enough to warrant a trip to the doctor's office and prescription drugs. You don't need to have complications in addition to the learning stage of breast-feeding.

Check with lactation consultants and information on the Internet to get help on any breast-feeding issues. I can't stress enough the importance of getting help. This will save you and your nipples, and you won't have to worry about whether your baby is getting enough milk.

## Pumping and Storing Breast Milk

Sometimes there are other factors involved and mum wants to pump because she needs to go back to work or just needs to be away from baby longer than the time between regular feeds. The La Leche League website offer tips on how to store milk, and so much more.

Think about this before you go and buy formula. Your breast milk is the perfect and nutritionally exact formula of vitamins, minerals and antibiotics exclusively for your baby. Formula can't even compete with this. Breast-fed babies, whether fed from the body or from a bottle of pumped milk, will be healthier with your immunities and will feel much more satisfied. Baby can easily digest breast milk, but may have a lot of trouble digesting manufactured substitutes.

Remember what goes in must come out—it is important to monitor your baby's urine and bowel movements, especially in the first few weeks. Continue to be aware as baby grows and develops, or you may find yourself with a baby that has an upset tummy and is expressing himself very loudly! If that happens, think back to what an older baby may have eaten, or to what mum may have eaten if nursing a newborn. Most women should be able to eat whatever they want. If a woman is used to eating it while pregnant, her baby will have a tolerance for it. Just watch when spicy foods are introduced into breast-feeding mum's diet as this may affect baby's tummy.

# Pacifiers

The choice to give baby a pacifier at birth is totally personal. Both sides of the pacifier dilemma have been explored extensively in literature and opinion. Personally, my children had pacifiers and they all breast-fed perfectly until I chose to wean them. None of them went to school with a pacifier; in fact, none of my children used a pacifier past the age of two years old.

I have talked with women that complain, "Baby won't leave me alone he wants to be on the breast *all* the time." Please take a moment to see if baby is feeding – does he making gulping noises and is his jaw moving in a constant sucking motion – or is he lounging at your breast and occasionally having a suck? If he is full because of his last feed and is not effectively nursing, then he just may be using you as a pacifier.

Women can often see their babies thumb-sucking in the ultrasound, and most notice babies putting hands or fingers into the mouth at birth. Babies receive joy and contentment from sucking. I say go buy the pacifier and let baby sleep while you get your sleep! It is essential for you to nap when baby naps, and using a pacifier maybe the way to achieve some much-needed rest. Overall, I am a firm believer that mums should listen to their instincts and make up their own minds on all decisions about their children.

*"The woman's choice itself may influence her
level of anxiety and apprehension, and in
obstetrics levels of anxiety have been shown
to predict obstetric complications."*
**Wiegers Study**

# The Indian Approach

Muneera, a lovely friend I have had the pleasure to
work with, is from India. She has written her own
beautiful birth story and the approach her culture has
to pregnancy and birth.

*In India, pregnancy is a sacred time for us women. A
woman carrying a baby is as special as perhaps a queen or a
goddess. She is, after all, a vessel for the creation of new life!
She will bring a child into the world. She must be protected
from all danger, every evil and any grief, fear or worry. Her
thoughts and feelings will become the baby she bears. Her
experiences and actions will shape the consciousness of this
new being. Her only purpose during this time is to nurture
her body and the baby, think beautiful thoughts and spend
as much time as possible in contemplation of the divine.
Every person around her will support her in this. She will be
cooked for, and allowed to rest with her legs elevated. She
will be treated to beautiful sights, sounds, smells, tastes and
sensations. She will be smothered with love so that she never
feels a moment of sadness. Her every desire is fulfilled
because it is seen as the child within speaking its needs. This
is the joy of childbearing as Indian traditions espouse and as
I experienced.*

*I live in Vancouver, Canada and since life is so different here, I adapted those traditions to my Western lifestyle. I worked for the first three months and then decided to stay home to enjoy my pregnancy. I gave myself the care that I would have otherwise received from my community in India. I cooked fresh food everyday and ate well. I loaded up on beneficial, alkaline, and energetically pure (sattvic) foods like milk, clarified butter (ghee), fruits and vegetables. I tried to tune into my baby, feel its every wish and satisfy its every craving. I refrained from any work too demanding on my new softening and quickly growing body. I gave myself warm oil massages and sang sweet songs to my belly. All of a sudden I could no longer watch movies that were suspenseful, violent or horrific. I lost my desire to read books and listen to music. Somehow, all I wanted was stillness and quiet. I respected that this was what was right for my baby, that they were her particular wants. And I gave thanks for the peace that I felt inside. It was as though all doubt about everything disappeared from my mind, and questions answered themselves before they were even asked. I felt within myself the power of the life-giving goddess.*

*Of course, there were also those moments when I felt like I was regressing back to my childhood. I wanted nothing more than to be held by my mother, and soothed by her healing touch. Especially so in my second and third month when I had strong nausea, and felt like something alien had usurped my body. I would phone my mama, all the way in India, and she would counsel me from ten thousand miles away. She told me how these were merely small tests and challenges to prepare me for my work as a mother. I felt comforted by her words and found a new strength for my* baby. Thankfully, by my second trimester, I felt the alien leave and my baby arrive. And then, all was bliss!

I would meet with my doula, and she would drop her little pearls of wisdom gently into my open hands. "Remember Muneera, you can give it all the treasures that you want, but all a baby really needs is love." Her words still echo in my mind and send surges of warmth through my body. This is the truest thing that anyone has ever said to me about child bearing.

### Mother and Daughter Relationship

We had planned for a home birth with midwives. My husband and I attended Jennifer-Lee's Birthing from Within prenatal classes and felt as prepared as we would ever be. Such classes are unheard of in India. Presumably, older women in the family and community prepare women for birthing in a more informal way. Unfortunately, all that tradition is lost in the "developed" areas of my country. In the city, we blindly trust in Western medicine practitioners who, in India, are often only out to make an extra buck. Modern hospital births are the norm, and Cesarean sections are a dime a dozen. The new wave of the return to empowered natural birthing has yet to wash over our cities. In the villages and rural areas, there is more traditional practice around birthing, but less and less each day.

In India, the tradition is for the woman to go to her mother's home for birthing and the first 40 days after. The idea is for her to be where she feels most at home, and where she has complete, loving care. Of course, underlying this tradition is the close bond shared between mother and daughter. We believe that new mothers need a kind of emotional support that only other women can provide. A husband may mean well, but he may not always be able to *fully understand what his wife really needs. With her mother, a girl is also safe from having to meet the sexual needs of her partner again before she is ready to. It also prevents the new father from becoming overwhelmed by the combination of the new baby and the emotional fragility of his partner. If the daughter cannot return home, often the mother will go and be with her daughter for the birth.*

*Of course, some of this may seem so absurd to people who come from a different worldview. I know that the success and utility of some of our customs hinge on the conservative and old-fashioned nature of gender roles and relationships. But that aside, I feel that there are still some truths that apply to every woman regardless of upbringing and culture.*

*In keeping with the Indian custom, my mother came to stay with us in Vancouver. We all squeezed into our little one bedroom apartment (as Indians regularly do). My mama happily slept out in the living room on my massage table. She coddled me wonderfully. I was ecstatic to be eating the comfort foods that I grew up with (and had dreamt of for the last nine months), that only my mama could prepare so perfectly. I was finally ready for the baby to arrive.*

*We went into labour early in the morning. It was 4 a.m. when I felt the first little uncomfortable cramping as I lay in bed beside James. I felt a bit sheepish for having gone to bed only at 2 a.m. the night before. After all my doula experience, and the many women I had advised to get good regular sleep in preparation for labour, I had stayed up late for the last few nights and was in a considerably sleep-deprived state for my own. I managed to sleep for a few hours, and awoke when I could no longer ignore the sensations in my belly. It was 8 a.m. My mama was outside, still asleep, when James and I woke her up with our excitedly grinning faces declaring the time had come.*

*Now for my mama, who had her babies during the time when birthing had become an industrialized process in the hospital – complete with pipes and tubes and big metal instruments – this whole "home birth in water" business was quite an outrageous idea. She definitely had her reservations about the whole thing. Well, she jumped to her feet and quickly made breakfast, after which she went into a corner of the apartment, laid down her prayer mat and started her prayers. She then continued to pray non-stop until the baby had been deposited safely into my arms. It is curious how the act of birthing in Indian cities has moved from the hands of the midwife (dai) into that of Western medicine doctors, but all the traditions that occur outside of the hospital have remained alive.*

*We laboured away the hours. James was the perfect birth partner. Loving, reassuring and steadying. I rocked in his arms, and walked around between contractions. My doula set up the birthing pool. The midwife arrived. It was noon. The contractions were now unbearable. I lost my center many times over, and started to doubt that I could do it. I was 5 cm dilated. The midwife offered to break the bag of waters sitting right at the cervix preventing the baby's head from pressing it open. I gladly agreed.*

*I sat in the pool for some semblance of a rest. The contractions now seemed back-to-back. I was no longer conscious of anything except my womb. I felt like I was in a hypnotic trance. My doula would stroke my third eye to help me focus. I went to a place that I have never even visited in my so-called morning meditations. James could no longer take away my pain or distract me. He was there, but on the outside. Oh, I was so glad he was there, but I knew that I had to finish the journey alone. It was now just my baby and me. I went for my last pre-motherhood pee. It was three in the afternoon.*

*As I leaned against the bathroom sink (the only time I ever did that without noticing how badly we needed to renovate our bathroom), I felt the desire to bear down. Oh, it felt so good to do that. My midwife slipped her hand inside and gave me the go ahead to do it. With every contraction, I would bend my knees, grab on really tight to the sink and push down. Then I was in the bedroom. I wonder how I got there, but I did. There was more of that low squatting. I was often on my knees too. I knew that I was screaming. In fact, the whole act of pushing out my baby felt like one long, loud, uncontrollable scream. I knew of nothing else—well, except maybe that my anus was going to pop right off my backside. Only from looking at the pictures later did I realize that James was with me, being my pillar as I rested in between pushes, holding and caressing me through it all. Then the midwife said that I had to lay down on the bed ... the baby's heartbeat ... something or the other. I panicked. And I said, "No, give me one more push." And out she came, one hand over her head (the little rascal), and she smiled at me.*

### Traditions of the Postpartum Period

*Then began the glorious postpartum period that I was so looking forward to. We Indians have an elaborate set of customs for after the baby is born. With each Indian sub-culture it differs slightly, but the underlying principles are the same.*

***Complete rest and warmth for mother for up to 40 days:*** *This confinement includes having someone to cook and clean for her, lots of help with the baby, a daily hot oil massage and bath, and as little activity as possible. Some women even bind the belly tightly with a cloth to help the muscles tighten. There is certainly no movement outside the house so as to protect mother and child from any unwanted external influences like cold, germs, negative energy, etc.*

***A special diet of warm, light and nourishing food:*** *Most people have a version of cream of wheat porridge that is eaten immediately after, especially for the first weeks. It is cooked with ghee (the most nourishing of fats according to Indians) and jaggery (gur- a dark, almost black, unprocessed cane sugar high in minerals and good for balancing hormones). Some other foods are milk, nuts and soupy* mung *beans.*

***Special herbs to rejuvenate reproductive organs, improve digestion, increase milk flow and reduce gas in both mother and baby:*** *There are some spices that we make into a tea and sip all through the day. My mother made me one with fennel seeds, ajwain seeds, fenugreek seeds and black pepper. I have heard other versions too. We also take herbs made into ball-shaped sweets or just plain in milk. Ginger in particular is believed to cleanse the uterus and control postpartum bleeding. I ate a spoonful of a dry mixture (made of dried coconut, dill, ajwain, poppy and sesame seeds, dried date and almonds) after meals to help my digestion and get good milk. We also use some dried herbs to insufflate the vagina to help it heal and tighten well.*

*I happily adhered to these customs as much as I possibly could because somewhere deep inside me I had faith that they were of value. I wished I could have had more massage, but I was happy with the occasional one I got (in India it is a lot more affordable to get a daily massage). I did massage on my baby everyday and still do at least once a week. She still loves it as much as she did when she was four days old. I know that the tea I drank saved me from many a long night with a fussing baby. She rarely got too uncomfortable from gas and when she did a simple tea made from roasted cumin seeds steeped in warm water quickly dispersed the bubble in her tummy.*

*My mother stayed with me and taught me everything I needed to know about a baby. She showed me how to bathe her, change her, wrap her up warm and tight and rock her to sleep. If I ever got too tired, my mama would take my little one and keep her outside so that I could sleep. I never reached a point of exhaustion while my mother was with me. I only realized how important that was for my state of mind when she once went away for a few days to visit a friend. I was left alone with a baby and a house to look after. I was so fatigued by the third day that I started to feel low. It is the only time I met the notorious postpartum blues. As soon as she returned the next day, and I rested myself again, I felt no trace of the sadness. I realized that good, supportive company during postpartum could really keep the blues at bay. She explained to me how women are in a fragile emotional and physical state after birthing. The hormonal changes that we go through demand special care. We must take the time to give ourselves the rest so that our bodies may return to their state of balance. The 40-day confinement made so much sense to me then.*

*Above all, my mother helped me transition into my new role as mother. She counseled me to surrender to my child, and to accept the changes that it brought into my life. She reminded me that it was normal to feel conflicting emotions of happiness and sorrow, intense love for baby yet resentment from the sacrifices I had to make, eagerness to be a perfect mother and frustration at not being able to control events and outcomes. I needed that gentle encouragement to let go of the way things were and open up to the joys that my child brought with her. I was so grateful for her wisdom and experience.*

### Indian Birth Ceremonies

*In every Indian sub-culture, the postpartum time is marked by several important ceremonies. There is much ritual attached to each event (the details of which would fill pages and pages yet so I will only describe them briefly here). For my family, the first one is on day six. It is the naming ceremony (the* chatti*). We gather with close family, food and gifts. The sister of the father names the baby by speaking the chosen name first into baby's ears and then out loud to the public. In most communities, the child is named only after consulting with an astrologer who creates the birth chart. He will appoint the letter (dictated by the birth planet of the baby) with which the name must begin.*

*The next ceremony is when we remove the baby's birth hair (the* aquiqa*). It is often only the first of many shavings. This is done on day 14 or 21. Special prayers and sacrifice accompany it. The custom of shaving the head is associated with benefits to the nervous and endocrine system of the child. It also makes for a beautifully thick crop of hair.*

*There are some other celebratory days that have been lost over the years in my family. Prenatally we would* celebrate the beginning of the seventh and ninth months with food and music. Postpartum, we would mark the last day of the woman's confinement, the first time a baby is placed in its cradle, the baby's first taste of weaning food, the appearance of the first tooth, the first time baby crawls on all fours, the piercing of the child's ears ... the list goes on and on. I love the festivities of birthing in my culture. It makes the journey into motherhood so much more enjoyable, and it brings the community closer together.

Then there is the business of the evil eye (**nazar**). Many people (including my Caucasian husband) laugh outright when I talk about it, but it is tremendously important to us Indians. We believe that there are negative energies out there that can cause harm to us, especially to our helpless babies. This evil eye can be cast by anyone, often without their even knowing it. Why, even a mother can cast it upon her own baby! So we take elaborate steps to avoid it. First, we put a black dot on the baby's head. This is said to draw the evil energy away from the baby by allowing it to rest on a perceived "imperfection." We also put on talismans and metal charms. In addition, we never praise the baby out loud, and say many prayers for its protection. If the evil eye falls on the baby, it gets sick. Then we undertake many rituals to remove it. I personally know people who use coconuts, knives, burning cloth, eggs, salt water and special crystals to name a few. I use a black string around my daughter's neck to ward against it.

When I look at the birthing experience I had, I feel wonder at what a complex combination of new and old it happened to be. I guess it is a reflection of how I myself am a mish-mash of traditional and modern. There are many customs that may sound like pure superstition to some. Yet, *even my scientific mind can accept them because energy and spirituality are a part of science in our tradition, and many of our beliefs are around maintaining positive energy and closeness to the divine. Then there are those customs that I choose not to follow, because they do not serve my beliefs and feel more like societal or religious limitations. In those instances, I opt for modern methods and ideologies. How wonderful to be able to choose from such a wealth of possibilities, to live in a time and place where that can be! I find it a beautiful combination that allows me to trust in my intuitive impulses and follow my heart. I try to have faith that I will be guided to do what is right, and hope to stay humble enough to learn the lessons that come my way.*

*This is my story. I know that many women have different experiences from mine, yet feel the same gratitude as I do because every experience of birth is special. Regardless of the cultural traditions, the process is the same. It is a miracle. It is our truest experience of God because it takes us to a place of such deep love. I hope that women always find the teachings that guide them easily through pregnancy, childbirth and after, and allow them to have that deeply spiritual experience.*

**Muneera Wallace, Doula, Mother,**
**Owner *www.inarasclothdiapers.com***

## Visualization or Hypnosis Birthing

This technique for labouring has hugely positive results and is one of the easiest tools I use—I only need my voice. I provide this technique all the time and I find that it is more effective if dad is involved, so I help to guide him in telling wonderful tales about specific moments that resonate with him and mum.

108

## Christie & Chava's Birth Story

I met this young couple at their summer home in downtown Vancouver; they live the other half of the year in Mexico where Chava is from. Christie wanted to be prepared for labour and delivery so she took two different prenatal classes. I had been hired specifically for Hypno-birthing, my spirituality, and because I am a Reiki Master. I am happy to do Reiki on a labouring mum. I may not utilize this often; it depends on what a woman wants and her belief system. Christie really wanted to have a water birth.

*Two days before her labour starts, Christie calls to tell me that she has mild cramping and she is feeling tired. The next night they go to visit friends, get home around midnight and go to bed.*

*Two hours later, a small gush of clear water wakes her. She calls and asks what she should do. I tell her we will wait until her contractions pick up and I advise her to try to get some rest.*

*4:45 a.m.: Christie and Chava phone to tell me they are going to the hospital to have her cervix checked. Good contractions have been constant for a couple of hours. Christie is very anxious to know how her cervix is dilating.*

*I arrive at the hospital and it is exceptionally busy. We have to wait for an assessment room. Finally at 5:45 a.m. Christie is checked and is only 1 cm dilated. Her cervix has thinned, but she is not being admitted. She asks for some pain management, and receives Morphine. This allows mum to rest and relax, and when relaxed, mum's cervix dilates quicker.*

*We have to wait a long time in the assessment cubicle. Mum has to deal with her contractions but being so tired her spirits are deflated. She is feeling frustrated because she was hoping she had progressed further. Finally the nurse comes in to administer the shot of Morphine. We get mum out of the hospital as quickly as possible and take her home to rest.*

*Mum tries to lie down on her bed but the lying position is uncomfortable. I suggest that she might want to try the tub. I fill the tub with warm water and put a pillow at the end so she can fully lay back to relax. Within the hour mum is out. She has no mobility in the small tub and the water cools too quickly. Filling another tub is beyond her tolerability at this point.*

*I try to help her get back into bed at 8:45 a.m. We had lots of pillows to prop her with and a hot water bottle on her back, but this does little to make her comfortable. She adjusts herself every few minutes and does not enjoy lying down. Mum is drowsy from the Morphine and has no energy to be upright or walking.*

*Mum tells us she might be sick. We scramble to get a bowl just in case. I notice mum has lots of bloody show. I ask her how she is feeling. Her contractions are slowly progressing and getting stronger and she has been managing well, but she just can't find a comfortable place to labour.*

*9:30 a.m.: Mum decides that she wants to go back to the hospital. She wants to talk to her midwife and have another cervical check done. We get mum dressed and put her in the car. I am riding in their car, and on the way back to hospital, Chava asks if I would like a coffee. He knows of a good place, and pulls a U-turn on a busy street and parks right up front of the coffee shop. I am thrilled at the chance to have a strong cup of coffee!*

At 9:50 a.m. we walk into the hospital and mum has a big gush of fluids. The fore waters may have broken earlier. She has some leaking, but this is probably the bag of waters. Although the hospital is still very busy, we manage to find our midwife. Ten minutes later Christie is checked and is 2-3 cm dilated. We decide to stay and walk the halls of the hospital.

At 10:45 a.m. Mum says she feels a big pressure. She can actually feel the baby moving down inside her. At 11:00 a.m. the obstetrician is supposed to come and check mum again, but it is so busy he won't be coming to see us at all.

We have been inside walking and we decide to go outside to enjoy the warm sunny summer day. The grounds of the hospital are like a park. After a couple of hours of walking we find a picnic table. Dad goes to his car to get a blanket and some drinks. Mum decides she wants me to try Reiki on her. I have done Reiki several times on labouring women and I am always amazed that when I put my hands close to their bodies and do Reiki, their contractions get stronger and closer. I really have to be mindful not to do this for too long. I do it intermittently. Mum and dad try talking to their baby. They try encouraging him to come, to please be born.

> Reiki is a healing modality, which is non-touch and similar to healing touch. It originated in Japan and has a delightful philosophy that one can live their life by. The motto, which I love, is:
>
> > Just for today, Do not worry.
> > Just for today, Do not anger.
> > Honor your parents, teachers, and elders
> > Earn your living honestly
> > Show gratitude to every living thing.

> *Reiki is a transfer of positive energy through the palm of one's hand, into and through the receiver. It is believed that the body has a natural ability to heal itself. The receiver, whose energy may be unbalanced, uses this natural universal energy to help the body, mind and spirit. My observation with the use of Reiki in labour is that it strengthens contractions, and it helps women relax. I only use this with permission from my labouring mum.*

The midwife finds us wandering through the assessment waiting room. She watches mum and then checks baby's heart rate with the portable fetal Doppler. The midwife tries to find us an assessment room, but the hospital is still crazy busy and there are simply no rooms available to us.

> *A fetal Doppler is a portable, hand-held heart rate monitor. It is used to listen to baby's heart beat and allows freedom from the stationary form of listening with bands around the belly while laying in bed for labouring mums. They have gotten popular as the general public can purchase or rent them. So pregnant mums are often listening at home to baby's heart beat any time they wish.*

Back outside we find a round table with space where mum can squat between the seats. When in the squat position she tells us she can feel the baby move down. The sensation is huge—she holds on to the seat and rocks.

1:00 p.m.: We go back inside. It's refreshing to come in from the heat every once in a while—the change of scenery. We don't walk very fast or very far; I am concerned that mum might faint. A nurse takes pity on us, *and gives Christie a birthing ball in an empty cubicle and allows to her sit.*

*This is just a crazy busy day for the hospital staff. There are lots of babies wanting to be born today! I continue to do Reiki on mum and I add in a shoulder massage. We have been massaging hips and back, which mum appreciates.*

*I wonder if the baby is facing posterior. I have seen harsh back labour, but this mum seems to be having a mild version, not that I would ever tell her that. Back pain is always difficult, and she is dealing with it very well.*

*1:20 p.m.: Finally there is a bed in the assessment room where we can have mum checked. She is 4 cm dilated, which is fabulous news because we can finally be admitted to a room. Mum really wants to be in the tub.*

*By 2:00 p.m. I have mum settled in a tub, and dad lays down for a nap. I sit beside mum on a stool and coach her through every contraction, always gently reminding her to breathe. I love to watch a woman in labour. The control and discipline that determined women show is amazing. She may be uncomfortable, she may feel lost and vulnerable, but this is all part of her journey into motherhood, and part of the reason it is so empowering for a woman to go through the birth process.*

*2:07 p.m.: Mum throws up. I wipe her and she settles back into the comfort of the tub. I put some music on in the room for her to relax with. Half an hour later the midwife comes in. She squats quietly in the bathroom and we both watch as mum gently sways in the tub on her back. Mum instinctually wants to be on her hands and knees. She turns over. I help. She sways forward and back and then mixes it with sideways swaying of the hips.*

*4:30 p.m.: The tub water has been re-warmed several times all the while mum is swaying her body. She finally decides to get out of the tub. We are drying mum and putting her onto the bed when dad wakes up.*

*4:46 p.m.: Mum is not comfortable in bed. After checking her blood pressure and having a listen to baby's heart beat, we suggest she get on the birthing ball.*

> The Birthing Ball is the same as an exercise ball in most gyms and work out establishments and also physiotherapist offices. Mum sits on the ball and rocks, allowing her hips to sway and for baby to ease his head into her pelvis.

*Mum is comfortable on the ball and has a bite of sandwich and a drink. The midwife comes back from another birth. She checks the cervix: mum is 5 cm dilated and a bit thinner.*

*At 5:30 p.m. mum asks for something for the back pain. She is given a sterile water injection in her back, then starts to walk around. This is four needles containing sterile water injected into four specific places on the back near the spine. It is quite effective in reducing some back pain.*

*6:15 p.m.: Mum makes the comment, "I don't want to be pregnant." It has been a long day and we still have a long night ahead of us.*

*6:40 p.m.: Mum is back in bed. There is a lot of swaying – standing – legs moving around, and then she says, "I can't do this." Five minutes later mum wants back into the tub. I hold the shower head on her while she gets in. She is swaying again back and forth and sideways on hands and knees in the tub.*

*7:10 p.m.: Mum gets out of tub and is checked— 5 cm dilated. The midwife goes to talk to the obstetrician on call. She inquires about starting Oxytocin. Mum returns to the tub.*

*8:25 p.m.: We help mum out of the tub. The midwife has been content allowing mum to go a bit longer, but now she checks her again—still 5 cm dilated.*

*I notice a difference in mum and ask her how she is feeling. She says there is no longer any back pain, but now it is lower down into her bottom. All her rocking in the tub has obviously helped baby to move into a different position. She is no longer having back labour.*

*8:55 p.m.: An I.V. is put into mum's hand and 20 minutes later Oxytocin is started. Mum is congested so I put some special "cold drops" for her sinuses on a tissue for her to inhale. This is a specialized formula for mums in labour.*

*10:30 p.m.: Mum is laying against a birthing ball on her knees on the bed then moves onto the floor on the ball to sit upright. Mum has been doing so well with the Oxytocin, managing her contractions very well.*

*10:45 p.m.: Mum is checked again and is 7-8 cm dilated and spines (the head has descended more in the pelvis) and baby is in a much better position. For the first time since this afternoon there has been significant progress. Mum is thrilled—we all are!*

*11:45 p.m.: Mum is checked again and is the same, but wants to push; she has had this sensation for the last three quarter hours.*

*12:10 a.m. Monday morning: There is a lot of bloody show and Christie has been having uncontrollable urges to push. She is checked again and is a fabulous 9.5 cm dilated with just a tiny bit of cervix.*

*12:30 a.m.: Mum is now 10 cm dilated and is starting to push. She is very strong and pushes well. Ten minutes into pushing we can see baby's head.*

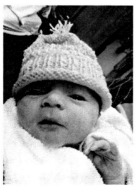

*1:14 a.m.: Only three quarters of an hour after Christie starts to push a beautiful baby boy is born. Mum has done a fabulous job of pushing her baby. Baby goes up onto mum's chest, skin-to-skin. Dad takes pictures. He so in awe of what has just happened, he is speaking very quickly in Spanish and mum is translating what he is saying to us. Dad speaks little English anyway, but with the sheer excitement of his son's birth it is simply too much for him to try.*

*1:35 a.m.: The placenta is delivered. Fifteen minutes later the midwife checks and there is only one small tear. The baby weights 8 lb 5 oz and he is very healthy.*

*3:00 a.m.: Breast-feeding went really well. Mum has some toast and tea, and everyone shows signs of getting ready for a nap. I decide to leave.*

This was going to be a water birth and for the most part Christie was in the water. The water certainly helped her manage her contractions, which resulted in no pain medication for the labour—something that she can always be proud of.

The water also had a profound outcome on this birth: had mum not turned baby while she was rocking in the water, she would definitely have had a Cesarean section. Again she proved to me that a driven woman in labour can achieve insurmountable odds.

# 5. Educating Dad

*"The knowledge of how to give birth without outside intervention lies deep within each woman. Successful childbirth depends on an acceptance of the process."*
**Suzanne Arms**

MOST MEN DO NOT READ PREGNANCY BOOKS or watch birth shows as often as their wives. They learn primarily from prenatal class, and prenatal visits with the doula. Doulas explain in detail how dads can help at the birth. With education we empower dads to be the best birth partners they can be. Dad's participation and attention to helping his wife navigate labour can create a deeper bond with mum than before. She can see and appreciate that dad helped her as she struggled through the birth process.

It thrills me to see dads wanting to catch their babies, and the care providers encouraging this. We are getting away from the scenario when dads waited down the hall to give out that cigar after hearing that his wife had delivered a girl or boy. Dad's emotional support and physical presence with mum is irreplaceable.

So what should dad expect when he brings his wife and baby home?

Life is consumed with mum trying to get enough sleep, breast-feeding and feeding herself. Mum should be allowed the first couple of weeks to recover from the birth and longer if she had a Cesarean section. Mum will be trying to schedule feedings, diaper changes and general household duties and she can quickly become exhausted. Having a simple chart that reminds busy parents when baby last fed, which breast he was on or when he last had a bowel movement or urinated may sound like so much, but at 3:00 a.m. it is easy to forget.

Mum will learn how to sit comfortably with a tender perineum, how to hold baby correctly and how to latch a baby even if he is fussy and ensure he gets a full feed. Your baby should want to feed every couple of hours and this can take time, so with the precious time in between it is important for mum to take care of her needs. Eating, bathing and napping can be a challenge and a struggle if she is trying to wash dishes and put clothes in the dryer.

One of the best things dads can do to help, is take some of the responsibility by co-ordinating with family and friends to bring cooked meals in, helping with doing the house cleaning or running errands for the first month. This allows mum the time to look after the high demands of a newborn.

A fabulous way for dad to have one-on-one bonding time with baby is to suggest that mum take some time to herself whether it is a nap, a tub or time away from the house. New babies usually stay up throughout the night and sleep during the day. This is very common and mum will work at changing this routine very quickly. Most babies are sleeping through the night by the sixth week home.

I suggest you encourage baby to stay awake during the day by talking to and playing with her. Then during evening feedings, keep the lights low, show her that she feeds and goes back to her bed. To help baby switch her routine, I suggest keeping the room quiet and dark, with only a night light on. Not too much stimulation like talk and play, but allowing baby to go right back to sleep with a cuddle or song. When she wakes during the day, do everything to keep her awake longer.

Using disposable diapers will allow her to sleep the night without having a wet diaper. I understand that more people are using cloth diapers. I used both when I had my babies. I chose to use disposables at night—there was too much precious sleep time lost getting up to change a wet diaper when my baby wasn't hungry.

Dad can help set up mum's special area for feeding baby and can keep it supplied with anything she might need. When she sits down to feed baby, dad might remind her to relax. It can be stressful in the beginning while she and baby are learning how to breast-feed. There may be concerns about whether baby is getting enough and mum may have nipple problems. Encourage her to get help if this occurs. Dad can take care of mum by listening to and responding to her needs and wants, making her daily life comfortable and easier and creating great family unity.

> "Birth is not only about making babies. Birth is about making mothers ... strong, competent, capable mothers who trust themselves and know their inner strength."
> **Barbara Katz Rothman**

## What Dads Might Need at the Hospital

There are some items dads should remember to pack in the hospital bag. Food – first and foremost, always have snacks that are easy to eat. Dads should make sure that the food they choose is free of obvious scent, if they will be eating in the room. The hospital may have a microwave oven for heating food. Mum's senses are on ultra alert, so she may cast dad from the room, as smells she can normally tolerate will make her tummy queasy.

Along with keeping mum hydrated, dad should remember to have his own beverages. I have seen some dads pass out from hunger, tiredness (or the site of blood and mum's bodily fluids). The hospital may have a kettle for instant tea or coffee. Dad may have a very long night and need something and the coffee shops and cafeteria will be closed.

A bathing suit or shorts is a good idea if you want to get into the tub or stand at the shower with mum. Most doulas encourage dad to stand next to mum when she is in the shower or birthing tub. If the tub is big enough, dad can get in with mum and cuddle up. Dad can also hold the shower nozzle and direct the spray onto mum's back or stomach, whichever feels better in the moment.

Have the camera and / or video camera ready to go with batteries fully charged (this is important) for when baby is coming. I have had lots of instances where dads get so wrapped up in the moment they have to be reminded that it is okay to start taking pictures. I keep my camera in my back pocket when I know we are getting close to delivery. Dad should have it close by when mum has gotten to 10 cm and is starting to push. It may still take two hours for her to push, but he will be ready.

When at the hospital, dads are encouraged to ask any and all questions that arise. There is never a question that is not important enough, and dad should always know what is happening and how his wife and baby are doing.

*"You knew just what to tell Joel, and he could tell me what I really needed to hear in labour."*
**Natasha**

## Baby Blues versus Postpartum Depression

It is common for a woman to have mood changes during pregnancy and especially after her baby is born. Her hormone levels started changing when she conceived, and postpartum her body is getting back to a more normal level. The combination of changes in her body, lack of sleep and concerns about the newborn can cause much anxiety for mum. She may also experience disruption of her eating and sleeping patterns, crying, sadness and lack of interest in intimacy. This mild form of postpartum depression which goes away in a few weeks, is called the "baby blues" and is easily treated with a healthy diet, regular exercise, spending quality time with dad or other moms, and taking moments for self-renewal whenever possible.

Most women will naturally struggle with becoming a new mum, especially for the first several weeks until a routine is in place. Postpartum depression can occur after delivery or up to a year later. The symptoms, just a few of which are disruptions in sleeping and eating patterns, feeling sad, hopeless or overwhelmed, and losing interest in activities she usually enjoys, last more than two weeks. If you notice anything different about your wife that would lead you to believe she might be suffering from this, please mention it to her care provider. It is better to talk to someone and get help than to allow your wife to suffer when she is not aware that this is happening.

## Scheduling Help

I was very impressed with this schedule, designed by a client that needed to have organization for a baby and a five-year-old. She had all the times filled in by volunteer family and friends and then she confirmed to everyone by emailing them a copy.

Your helpers may bring cooked dinner or may come and cook, do the household chores, take a sibling to and from school or activities, allow you to nap or have time to be with baby.

| | | Sun date | Mon | Tue | Wed | Thu | Fri | Sat |
|---|---|---|---|---|---|---|---|---|
| Morning | | | | | | | | |
| | | | | | | | | |
| Afternoon | | Sally to Park | | | | | | |
| | | **Grandma** | | | | | | |
| Dinner | | | | Bringing Pizza | | Cooking Steaks | | |
| | | | | **Michael** | | **Michael** | | |
| Bedtime | | | | | | | | |
| | | | | | | | | |

## Darlene and Chris's Birth

I sit and reflect on the birth I just attended, and realize that sometimes all a doula needs to do is be present and talk gently to a labouring woman.

*I am called to attend the birth of a couple in their thirties, first baby, both are very excited. It is her due date. About 5% of women go into to labour and delivery on their due dates. It also happened to be my son's birthday, so I knew this new baby would be exceptional!*

*It is the afternoon and Darlene says she is in labour. Her mucus plug came out earlier that morning and she has been having mild contractions since, but nothing regular.*

*At 5:20 p.m. her contractions are coming closer together and are now longer. At 7:00 p.m. Chris calls, frantic, and asks if I could please come. The contractions are coming every four minutes and lasting two minutes. I get ready to jump in my car when Chris calls back. He has given me the wrong buzzer number for their apartment. I laugh and start my drive. It brings joy to my heart when I hear that kind excitement in someone.*

*After I arrive and ask a few questions about contractions, I see that Darlene looks like she has progressed further than she knows. I ask, "Can you feel anything in your bottom?"*

*"Yes," she says. "I feel like I want to poo."*

*I call the care provider to tell her that we are on our way to the hospital.*

*Chris follows my car. I think he wants a little help focusing on where to go. As we come up to red lights and stop, I can see in my rear view mirror that Darlene is not* managing well, and Chris's frantic look is worrying me. We drive a bit faster; thankfully it is a short drive to the hospital.

The care provider is not there yet. The nurse tells us to wait because they have to clean one of the assessment rooms first. After the next contraction, Darlene quietly tells us that she wants to poo. I turned to the nurse and firmly tell her we need a room—she wants to push!

We are promptly directed to the smallest assessment room; it is the only one clean. The nurse checks mum, who is 9 cm dilated. The nurse races out to tell the charge nurse and within five minutes we have a wheel chair and a nurse that takes us up to our room.

I immediately run a tub of water for Darlene. She is a bit out of control, partly because of the news about her progress; she is also overwhelmed by the moment, and by not knowing what she wants or needs.

In the tub she feels fabulous. We get her something to drink, and I try to calm her. She asks for drugs. In my interview she told me that she thought she wouldn't handle pain well and fully expected to have an epidural.

The nurse brings her the portable gas to try. It doesn't help, but I am thinking Darlene must be 10 cm dilated and ready to push. I go out to get the midwife, and ask if she can reassess.

9:03 p.m.: Just two hours after I am called to the house, Darlene is told she is 10 cm dilated and can push. Panic! She wants the epidural, and is crying because she doesn't know what to do. Chris and I calm her down. I tell her she is a strong woman and she can do this. Darlene is worried that she doesn't know what to do. I tell her to listen to her body and do what she feels her body wants, which includes moving, swaying and vocal noises.

We try to put Darlene on the bed, and then we move her to a standing position beside the bed. Darlene is still asking for the epidural until her water breaks. Then it is like a light goes on in her mind. She realizes that she has progressed and she starts to work with her contractions.

Darlene squats and makes deep guttural noises and pushes into her bottom with the contraction. We put her on the bed because her legs are tired. She is squatting again and then moves onto her back.

At 10:38 p.m. Chris is instructed to move away from Darlene's side to the end of the bed so he can catch his beautiful baby boy. Darlene has had no drugs, has pushed less than an hour and half, and her placenta is delivered five minutes after the baby.

Keaton breast-feeds after Darlene and Chris have their time to look at and talk to him and everyone is settled in nicely by midnight.

The whirlwind birth, as exciting as it was, left me thinking, "I didn't do much today." However when I take my leave and mum says, "I couldn't have done it without you" and follows up with, "it was when, in every contraction, you put your head next to mine and gently whispered your instruction."

I would tell her when to take a breath, when to push and when to relax, encouraging her to listen to her body.

Chris was beside her the whole time, always calling her endearing names, caressing her, kissing her and doing everything and anything he could to help keep her comfortable. It was a loving birth.

Darlene realized that with her quick birth, and the fast dilation of the cervix and quick progression of the labour, that you do not have the time to grow into your next phase. Everything was done quickly and it can be overwhelming for women. Darlene listened and trusted when Chris and I said, "Listen to your body," "You can, and are, doing this."

Now Darlene knows how strong of a woman she really is.

*THE HUMAN TOUCH*
*'Tis the human touch in this world that counts,*
*The touch of your hand and mine,*
*Which means far more than to the fainting heart*
*Than shelter and bread and wine;*
*For shelter is gone when the night is o'er,*
*And bread lasts only a day*
*But the touch of the hand and the sound of the voice*
*Sing on in the soul always.*
**Spencer Michael Free**

# What to Take to the Hospital

### Labour and Delivery

Here are some ideas of items to pack in your bag for labour and delivery. This is just an outline of the basics. Please feel free to add or delete to suit your individual needs and experience.

- Labour Aid (see further for the recipe)
- Light snacks, possibly grapes, blueberries (frozen), Popsicles
- Snacks & drinks for dad
- Birth Ball
- Lip balm
- Shorts/bathing suit for dad – if he is going to be in the tub or standing at the side of shower with the shower nozzle
- Camera, video camera with fully charged batteries and extra film
- Aromatherapy items – put the scent on a handkerchief and in a plastic locking baggie
- CDs, music on computer, iPod
- Pictures of wedding, children, pets, any visualizing tools – these can be on a computer or in an album or picture frame
- Pillows – cover with several pillow cases that can be thrown out when birth is over, as they may get soiled

## Items for After the Birth

- Housecoat and slippers
- Personal items – pads, shampoo, vitamins, toothbrush, toothpaste, contact lens solution, deodorant, etc.
- Change of clothes for mum to go home in
- Outfit for baby to go home in

- Blanket to cover baby
- Diapers for baby
- Car seat for baby
- Change of clothes for dad, and any personal items if staying overnight
- If having a vaginal birth, snacks and drinks for both mum and dad, take out food may be brought into most hospital rooms
- If Cesarean birth, you will be on an easily digested soft foods diet. Digestive cookies (they have molasses in them) are very good to help get your system started after the drugs and surgery

*"Women's bodies have near-perfect knowledge of childbirth; it's when their brains get involved that things can go wrong."*
**Peggy Vincent**

## Labour Aid Recipe

Here is the recipe for Labour Aid. Use in active labour to keep mum's energy up when she no longer wishes to eat. Giving her nutritious fluids is essential.

In a blender, mix:

- 1/3 cup fresh lemon or cranberry juice
- 1/3 cup honey (to taste)
- 1/4 tsp salt
- 2 crushed calcium/magnesium tablets (blend of vitamin), or liquid form
- water to make 4 cups

Mix well and freeze.

- Honey is for calories: fuel for the body
- Salt keeps the electrolytes balanced through the hard work of labour
- Calcium/magnesium feeds hard-working muscles
- Water hydrates
- Lemon or cranberry for flavor

Mix up a batch ahead of time just before your due date. Freeze it in small ice cube trays, then put the cubes in a Ziploc freezer bag. If you want to make Popsicles, do so preferably in dripless containers. This allows mom to walk around without fear of a mess. Make the drink to the mum's taste. Flavors often seem stronger to women in labour. The cubes can be put into a drinking container (preferably with a straw) only a few at a time and diluted with water to make it more palatable. The bag of cubes is easier to transport to hospital than jars or jugs of liquid. Put your name on the bag and put the bag in the freezer at the hospital when arriving.

## Home Birth – Water Birth

In this book I have described hospital births. This is where most women labour and deliver their babies. I admit I work primarily at the hospital. I have, however, attended home births and they are the best, most comfortable places a woman can have her baby.

If you are looking for a water birth, candles, variety of music, no restrictions, a gentle environment, a midwife and an endless list of advantages, home births have everything going for them. You hire your midwife, prepare and have an amazing time labouring in your own home and sleeping in your own bed that evening.

My next story shows that labouring at home means you can enjoy your own comforts, loudness of music, having candles everywhere, filling the tub so you can slide in or come out at your leisure and eating and drinking what you want with no restriction. Home is a gentle place where a midwife can delicately bring a baby into this world.

I prefer home births because there are no charts to be written on, no time lines to be followed, the environment is not sterile or medical like hospital—just a totally relaxed environment. Sometimes more family members help out and it truly feels like a "birth" day celebration.

The midwife always has her back-up plan if anything goes awry. She has privileges at a hospital close by and an ambulance can be there to take you to hospital if that is needed. The bad stories get circulated faster than the wonderful pleasant home birth stories.

Just remember that this is a viable option for birth.

> *"Natural childbirth allows the hormones that have been working for women for thousands of years to fulfill their functions. This is more important than just helping a woman through labor and delivery. Birth-related hormones also affect well-being much later in life."*
> **Janet Schwegel, *Adventures in Natural Childbirth***

## Danielle and Dave's Birth Story

*I first met with this couple four months before their due date. I chose this story for this chapter about dads because Dave was such an amazing birth partner, husband and dad. Dave was so responsible for the care of Danielle and his baby, and the love I witnessed from this man for his family was simply beautiful.*

*Danielle and Dave are artistic young people. They designed and painted a wall-to-wall, ceiling-to-floor sized Dr. Seuss design on two walls in the baby's room. It makes you feel like you are in "Whoville."*

*They have a midwife. The birthing tub has been rented for a month (two weeks before and two weeks after their due date) and they are excited about having a water birth at home.*

*It is six days past Danielle's due date. The baby is in the perfect position for birth and is moving a lot. Mum has been asked to go in and have the traditional monitoring and stress testing done in the next day if labour has not started.*

*The next morning Danielle is asked to take the "midwifery concoction" recipe; it is usually successful at helping labour begin. Funny, when most women are "threatened" with tests and drinking concoctions (or a booked C-section) the body miraculously seems to start the natural process of labour.*

*It is 11:30 p.m. and mum loses the mucus plug and has lots of bloody show. Her contractions start and are approximately eight minutes apart and are lasting 15 to 20 seconds.*

*4:45 a.m.: I am called to come to the house. I arrive and Grandma Betty and Dave are both up helping and supporting Danielle. A half hour after I arrive, Danielle's contractions are about seven minutes apart. She is hungry so we give her tea and a granola bar. We are standing in the kitchen with a cup of tea watching as she moves around swaying her hips every time a contraction comes.*

*5:40 a.m.: Contractions are starting to space out a bit. This seems like early labour and I worry everything will stop. We have Danielle walk around and I have conversation with her through each contraction. Betty has put on chicken soup—I am told that this is a must in Jewish households. Not only is it good for colds, but it is beneficial to labouring women. The smell is heavenly!*

*7:15 a.m.: The contractions slow right down and are sporadic. I leave to go home for awhile. I ask Danielle to get some rest. Both she and Dave lay down to take a nap.*

*11:45 a.m.: I get a call to come back to the house. Danielle's contractions are still not regular, but she has had one that was three minutes long and is having a hard time concentrating through them, so they both want me for support. In my nap I had a fascinating dream. I envision a grandma figure, wearing a dark green dress and holding a little boy's hand. I was intrigued but didn't quite know what it meant.*

*12:25 p.m.: Danielle is lying downstairs cuddling with Dave and listening to music when I arrive. The midwife has been called and will be here within the hour to check on Danielle's progress. We help bring Danielle upstairs to put her in the birthing pool for some relief. She is very hot from her body working hard all night.*

*Danielle asks that we light all the beeswax candles for the birth. When all the candles are lit we comment on how calm the lighting is in the room and the smell is very soothing.*

*1:03 p.m.: Danielle tells us she wants to push. I ask her to breathe through her contractions. I suggest that she get out of the tub and sit on the toilet; it has been awhile since she was there. However sitting there she really feels the pushing urge and we see lots of bloody show.*

*The midwife shows up so we take Danielle into her bedroom to lay down.*

*1:38 p.m.: Everyone is very excited finding out that Danielle's cervix is 7-8 cm dilated. Dave decides to get into the tub with her and we are listening to some fabulous music. There is such ambiance, candles only lighting the house, the curtains in the living room where the tub is have been closed for privacy. The feeling is of love and peace in the room. Dave tells us about "Bear" and what it has meant in his life and how he believes it is one of his animal guides.*

*Later when I go home I read in my "Power Animal Oracle Cards" (by Steven Farmer) what this animal means. Bear is described as:*

> "Boundaries ... Stand your ground ... be your complete self – the self that the Creator wants you to be and that you know in your heart of hearts is your destiny – you must not only define who you are, but also who you are not. It's only when you can say a clear "No" that you can say a clear "Yes," and both are equally important in defining where your edges are.
>
> Setting your boundaries in this way increases your confidence and sense of autonomy, and your choices become much clearer. This doesn't mean to always say "No"; it just means to be secure in knowing that you can. This is critical in accomplishing your mission, whatever that may be.

> Come from strong love, without malice or aggression, and let them see and feel your full presence. It will work every time. Protection. Creativity. Solitude. Healing."

*2:22 p.m.: The midwife checks Danielle's cervix while she is in the pool. There is only the last edge of cervix to go. Dave is rubbing her back while squatting behind her. Betty has been floating around outside the room, peaking in and not wanting to be a distraction. She quietly gets us towels and drinks for Danielle and Dave. She even takes the dog for a walk.*

*2:30 p.m.: Danielle tells us she wants to push.*

*2:40 p.m.: We help Danielle out of pool. She walks into the kitchen – she immediately goes onto hands & knees – she can't walk, only crawl. She wants to go to her bedroom; she wants her bed. Her contractions have intensified out of the pool.*

*3:00 p.m. Danielle gets back into the pool for some relief. The water is incredibly soothing. While sitting beside the tub I ask Danielle who the woman in the picture is. She tells me that it's her grandma who had just passed away about six weeks previously. I tuck this information away for now.*

*3:38 p.m.: Danielle is going back onto her bed. The midwife does a quick check. There is still a tiny bit more cervix to go. She easily pushes this back when Danielle has a contraction. The midwife says she wants to break Danielle's waters.*

*4:16 p.m.: Danielle starts to push and progress is going well—we change and get her up to pee and sit on toilet for a few contractions.*

*4:30 p.m.: The second midwife arrives to help with the birth. Many midwives work with a second pair of hands.*

*4:50 p.m.: Danielle is tired of sitting on the toilet and goes back to the tub. She can concentrate well and has lots of energy for pushing. She is trying all different positions, hands and knees, lots of movement to the soothing music.*

*6:00 p.m.: Danielle goes back to her bed. She has difficulty finding the best position. She tries her back, hands & knees, side lying ...*

*6:55 p.m.: We suggest she try pushing on the toilet. Dave gets behind her on the toilet and is bracing her, holding her upright as she is pushing. The midwives take a break and leave Dave and I to cheer Danielle on—she is working hard and starting to progress nicely. Having just us in the room seems to have made a huge difference for Danielle's progress.*

> *When women sit with their legs apart or slightly leaning forward, gravity gives baby the best chance to position himself in a good anterior position as he faces the back of mum's pelvis. At the pushing stage sitting on a toilet allows for this position. It is very comfortable as there is no pressure on her perineum or bottom — visually we see great progress.*

*The bathroom is extremely small, approximately 3 x 4 ft. As Danielle gets closer, the midwife and I trade spots. We have Dave, two midwives and myself squatting in front of Danielle on the floor. The baby has started to crown, the midwife contorts her body to reach down to grab baby.*

*7:41 p.m.: Danielle delivers sitting on the toilet. The midwife gets Dave to reach over and cut the cord. She hands the baby to the other midwife who is waiting with a warm blanket to take him to the bedroom. We get Danielle off the toilet and Dave stretches.*

*We place Danielle onto her bed and at 7:52 p.m. the placenta is delivered. Roland is placed on Danielle's chest, skin-to-skin, and the midwife checks to see if stitches are needed. Danielle is going to need a couple so the midwife attends to that. The baby is weighed and is 7 lbs. 5 oz. and, of course, perfect.*

*We put Roland to the breast and he starts nuzzling and sucking on the nipple, he gets to suck 25 minutes each side.*

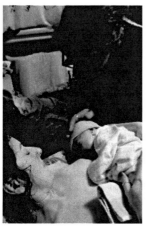

*I explain to Danielle about my dream from this morning. I saw a woman in the same green dress—in my dream that was the picture of her grandma. She was standing and holding a little boy's hand. They both watched us, as his soul was waiting to enter his little boy's body. Danielle is thankful for the story about her grandma as she's been upset that her grandma passed away before the birth.*

*9:20 p.m.: I help Danielle as she gets up to have a shower. We rewrap Roland, put clean sheets on the bed and then Betty brings in some chicken soup and something to drink for Danielle. We have all been commenting all day how wonderful the subtle scent simmering in the kitchen was.*

*10:00 p.m.: I am given a sandwich and bowl of delicious chicken soup, then leave Danielle, Dave and Roland snuggled together in bed.*

A special thanks and hug to Betty for all her help and her excellent cooking. Dave was fabulous support for Danielle. It's so wonderful to watch a strong woman birth her baby with a great team.

I found this to be a very special, spiritual birth.

# 6. Common Questions

*"People never sing ... except in the bathroom. Birthing women also make their natural sounds next to running bath water. There is something about the power of water. People are drawn to water, spas, and sacred streams. Women in labor are drawn to water, too."*
**Michel Odent, MD**

As you get closer to your exciting "birth" day, you may feel apprehensive and thrilled about your little angel's arrival. Your body has been changing, especially in the last four weeks leading up to labour. Hormones are being released throughout your body relaxing your muscles and ligaments. You may have noticed that your emotions are all over the place and you are more tired than usual. Some women have a nesting period just before birth where they go crazy cleaning their homes in preparation.

I am always being asked, "When will labour start and how will it progress?" Here are some common questions and useful suggestions about that fabulous day, but I remind you to always discuss with your care provider for the best clarification.

# Before Labour

Should I take vitamins when pregnant?

- Prenatal vitamins are recommended by your care provider.

- Take folic acid, usually found in prenatal vitamins, when trying to get pregnant. Folic acid helps with brain and spinal cord development.

- Eating whole leafy foods can only give some of what a developing baby will need.

What is the difference between a midwife and a doula?

- You have a midwife or doctor look after you through prenatal, labour and postpartum care— they will catch your baby and perform all clinical duties.

- A doula is a non-clinical, professional birth coach.

I heard I can help ripen my cervix before labour. Is this true?

- There are many teas you can drink; health food stores and your care provider can give you the information regarding what works best.

- There are a lot of books containing information about natural approaches to labour and child birth. One that comes to mind is by Susun S. Weed called, *Wise Woman Herbal for the Childbearing Year.*

Can I do anything to prepare my body for labour?

- Sit and rock on a birthing ball several times a week.
- Perineal massage.
- Take very good care of yourself, including body massages, sleep, proper eating and staying calm.
- Go on your last few dates before baby and babysitters.

What can I do to prevent back labour?

- You want an Occiput Anterior positioned baby when you go into labour, meaning you can rub baby's spine on the outside of your belly.
- You might try being mindful when sitting, to watch your posture. In the last month, be aware to sit forward with your legs spread wide apart as much as is comfortable. This gives the heaviest part of baby, his head, the gravity to slide to a forward position in your belly.

What is perineal massage?

- This helps soften and relax the tissue where baby's head will stretch at birth.
- Use natural oil.
- Lay down in a warm tub or your bed – relax and be comfortable.
- *Gently* massage the tissue on the perineum.

What is an induction cocktail?

- Traditionally midwives have used herbs to help pregnant women.
- To help induce labour there is a mixture that you can make and drink.

- Please ask your care provider if and when you might be able to take this.

What can I take for morning sickness?

- Soda crackers and more soda crackers.
- Fresh ginger root.
- Fennel seeds: you can make them into a tea.
- Always check with your care provider, and look for teas in health food and homeopathic stores.

What can I do to help me sleep at night?

- The last month of pregnancy is tough – use a lot of pillows to prop your growing tummy.
- Be good to yourself, have warm relaxing tubs, have your partner give you a massage, listen to relaxing music.
- As tough as it is, it will be over soon – think of it as Mother Nature preparing you for breast-feeding every few hours.
- Going to bed early and getting rest the weeks leading up to the birth can make a huge difference when you are in labour and you start your birthing marathon.

How do I get rid of heartburn?

- Acid reflux and indigestion are common in pregnancy. Sometimes caused by hormone changes in your body, watch what you are eating as you get further along in your pregnancy.
- Your baby can push his legs into your stomach and can cause the acids to push into your esophagus.

- Try eating small meals more often during the day.
- Avoid spicy or fatty foods. Milk and yoghurt can help.
- Stop eating at least one hour before you go to bed at night. Ask your care provider for help.

How will I know I am in labour?

- There are lots of signs – ask your care provider or doula.
- Most women have Braxton Hicks contractions, which are common leading up to labour. Women tell me "the contractions have changed." It is hard to describe the difference, but you will notice it.
- Your water may break.
- You may lose the mucus plug.

When should I call the care provider or my doula when I am in labour?

- They both like a call when you think you might be in early labour. They can guide you from there. Possibly you may be given suggestions on how to encourage labour or if it is in the middle of the night, how to relax and have a nap before labour really kicks in.

Should I call my care provider or hospital in the middle of the night if I am in labour?

- Yes, definitely. Talk to and have a plan with your care provider about this.

How many people can I have in the delivery room with me?

- Please ask your care provider about having family and friends in addition to your support.
- If the delivery is at the hospital they may have a restriction.

What is electronic fetal monitoring?

- The care provider wants to listen and monitor baby's heart rate.
- They will lay you in a bed, put bands around your tummy and you are asked not to move around. A machine sends out a paper tracing of the heart rate and contractions.
- This is common in high-risk and overdue pregnancies, but ask your care provider this great question so you can understand the reasoning behind it.

What is a Doppler and can I use this instead of the constant electronic fetal monitoring for more mobility?

- A Doppler is a portable, non-invasive ultrasound machine that monitors blood flow and blood pressure.
- The nurses can use the Doppler on your belly every fifteen minutes and this allows you greater mobility if you want to walk around or get into a tub or shower.
- Women with low-risk pregnancies often have this type of monitoring.

What to do with a head cold or illness when still pregnant?

- Take good care of yourself with proper rest, nutrition and sleep.

- There are some homeopathic, natural tinctures that you can use—ask a professional about this.

When can I go into labour, when is the best time to head to the hospital?

- Follow the 4-1-1 rule: When contractions are four minutes apart, one minute long and continuous for one hour.

- You will go through different stages with many changes in labour. Try and stay at home as long as you can. Home is a more comfortable place to be labouring than in hospital.

Why do I need to drink so much in labour?

- Think of your body as running a marathon—the desire diminishes as you progress through your labour, but you definitely need to replenish fluids that your body uses.

What happens if my baby is breech?

- Some doctors may allow a breech delivery; look in your area for someone who does.

- Before labour starts try Webster's Chiropractic Technique—lots of hands and knees and rocking, cold and hot, swimming and hand stands in water, lying head down on a board that is on an angle.

- Please check with your care provider.

What can I expect for pain relief?

- Typical in my city, women start with Entinox or nitrous oxide. This takes the harshest part of the contraction away, but you will still feel the contractions.

- Sterile water injections can be given for back labour pain. The care provider will inject needles into your back in four areas – note that it does sting.

- There are many more options to consider for pain relief, depending on your scenario. Consult with your care giver.

- Your doula should have some natural ways to help.

- As a last option, the epidural takes away all pain, but you no longer have mobility and you run the risk of contractions slowing down.

- You will need Oxytocin to augment or increase the contractions again. This is where I.V.s are started and you become confined to the bed.

- Your doula will know what is routinely given in your particular area.

Try and remember to take good care of yourself. As you get close to your due date, go on your last date nights together, and above all try and nap when you feel the need, and try to stay calm and relaxed.

## Labour

I'm not sure what to expect in labour.

- Every labour is different. Find a good doula or support person and go over all the scenarios.

- A doula can spend a prenatal visit talking about and answering questions. The conversation should be specific to you and your concerns.

What happens when I lose the mucus plug?

- It is an indication that your body is getting ready to go into labour, however labour may start right away, or within hours or within the next two weeks.

What does the mucus plug look like?

- The mucus plug is a white, creamy, clear, slimy substance usually with a small pink or brown tinge, similar to snot or a jelly fish. Once dislodged you should experience more slimy discharge. If any other colors appear please contact your care provider right away.

What is the dark discharge that I have?

- Your baby may have had a bowel movement and the substance is meconium. The color is dark brown or dark green, and your care provider needs to be aware of this right away.

Am I going to throw up in labour?

- Some women throw up. The hormones released in active labour can make you throw up. This is normal. When you are further along in your labour, it usually helps to dilate you more, sometimes a full centimetre. (I get excited when a woman throws up.)

Should I only push when I have a contraction?

- Yes, only push with the contraction, and use every bit of it. You want to work with your body and you need the time in between contractions to rest, some women even take a quick nap, and that may be only twenty seconds.

Can I push before I am 10 cm dilated?

- No! If and when you get the urge to push, make sure that the care provider checks that your cervix is 10 cm dilated. If you push too early your cervix may swell, and then you will have to wait for it to return to normal.

I heard I can breathe through the pushing stage?

- I have seen lots of women for various reasons breathe and grunt their way through the pushing stage. It is something to talk to your care provider about and ask your doula.

Will you help give me direction with positioning when I am ready to push?

- Yes, definitely. This is a big part of what your doula can do for you.

Do you give perineal massage or warm compresses when baby is crowning?

- Ask the care provider if they do this. A doula does not touch this area. Perineal massage helps stretch the area, and hopefully can help prevent or reduce tearing or the need for an episiotomy.

What is the difference between episiotomy and a tear?

- An episiotomy is a surgical cut made to the perineum to enlarge the vaginal opening to accommodate the delivery. A tear occurs when the skin tears naturally in response to delivery. Ask your care provider for literature that describes recovery time, pain factor, risk of infection and risk of complications for each method.

What are forceps and why might I need to use them?

- For a baby that has a big head and is having difficulty coming through the pelvis, sometimes forceps are needed—ask your care provider.

- The "Kiwi," a vacuum-assisted delivery device, is also used in this way. It is a round cup applied to the baby's head with suction. The care provider may use this to help baby come under the pelvic bone.

Can I expect to see my care provider during labour or just for the birth?

- Some care providers will show up at the end of your labour or they may not be in to see you very often. This is a huge reason you should consider having a doula. We provide constant care and stay with you during labour. We can help you to navigate your way through all the changes you will experience.

An interesting observation – though definitely not scientific – I notice lots of my clients, while pushing, have beautiful pedicures. I wonder what the correlation between a relaxing day at the spa and going into labour is all about?

# After Baby is Born

How often do I have to breast-feed my new baby?

- Breast-feed baby every two to three hours. When your milk comes in, feed when baby is hungry.

Baby is sleepy and doesn't want to eat. Is that normal?

- No, this is not normal. You should consult with your care provider or a lactation consultant.

Can we take pictures and / or video tape our birth?

- At my hospital clients are encouraged to take pictures or video tape any and all of the birth. Check with your care provider and hospital protocol.

Can my husband help catch my baby or can he cut the cord?

- At my hospital and with the SCBP care providers dads are encouraged to participate at the birth. Check with your care provider.

When do you clamp and cut the cord?

- There is much research and more discussion on the benefits of cutting the cord before or after it stops pulsing. Read more about this, and ask your care provider their philosophy.

When the cord dries and falls off can we have an "innie"?

- I get this question so many times I include it here – you simply have to wait for the cord to dry and fall off. There is nothing you can do to make it an "innie". Sorry.

Will my baby have to go directly to the bassinette for the nurses and doctors to check her vitals or can she come directly to my chest, skin-to-skin?

- Yes, definitely, but discuss with your care provider any circumstances under which this would not happen.

Can the eye ointment be delayed for an hour? Or not given at all?

- The eye ointment is optional in some jurisdictions. Ask your care provider about all of the options and reasons.

Should I have my son circumcised?

- This procedure used to be standard practice, but is now done at a later date by a specialist. Read all of the research and discuss the options with your care provider.

If a Cesarean section has occurred and mum is in recovery and away from baby, then dad can step in and cuddle baby skin-to-skin. This can be a very special bonding time with baby until mum is available to start breast-feeding.

The breast is all a baby needs in the beginning first few hours. Babies do not need to eat anything extra—instinctually they go to the breast.

# At Home

Why does baby sleep all day and stay up all night?

- A newborn's sleep cycles are based around the need to eat frequently. This is why they can wake up three to ten times a night. A newborn actually sleeps twice as much as an adult, but half of that time is in the day when it is less noticeable to busy parents. This is a natural cycle, and parents should wait at least six weeks before trying to instil a sleep schedule. Gradually the baby's routine will change as he learns from mum and dad that daytime is for fun and night time is for quiet.

How do I bathe my new baby?

- The nurses in the hospital show you how to give your baby a bath before you leave. If you are not sure ask for help. Keep baby warm by wrapping her in a towel and washing her head first, pat dry, then put her into the small bathing tub and wash. Baby can be washed on the counter with a cloth if she is really fussy in a tub.

How often do I bathe baby?

- Babies don't get dirty, so it isn't necessary to bathe them every day. Use your own discretion. Keep their bottoms clean with wipes or a clean face towel, and use diaper cream if you see a rash.

What can I use on baby's skin?

- Water is usually enough. Soap can dry her skin. You may try natural or mild products so as not to irritate her skin.

How do I store my breast milk?

- Breast milk at room temperature will last:
  - 24 hours at 15 degrees C
  - 10 hours at 19 to 22 degrees C
  - Four to six hours at 25 degrees C
  - Four hours at 30 to 38 degrees C
- In a refrigerator:
  - Eight days at 0 to 4 degrees C
- In a freezer:
  - Two weeks in the freezer compartment in your refrigerator
  - Three to four months in a self-contained freezer of a refrigerator
  - Six months or longer in a separate deep freeze that is constant at -19 degrees C
- Look up the full information on LeLeche League's Canadian website *www.lllc.ca*, the U.S. website *www.lllusa.org*, or the international site *www.llli.org*.

When can I give my baby a bottle without confusing him/her?

- The magic time is six weeks. Baby should have an established breast-feeding routine by then. If she gets a bottle too early she may prefer that. Bottles are easier to suck from and she may not want to go back to the breast. For whatever reason, if you are having a struggle, ask for help. You can usually get her back on the breast.

Why is it so hard to burp my breast-fed baby?

- Breast-fed babies don't take in much or any air when they feed. It may not be as necessary to burp baby.

- Rubbing baby's back is also very affective in getting her to burp.

My baby won't/doesn't want to feed in public and is fussy. Why?

- It could be partly because you aren't as physically comfortable where you and baby are sitting, or psychologically it is uncomfortable for you and the baby is picking up on that stress.

Why is baby fussy?

- Check the diaper. Is baby tired or hungry? If these three things are fine, then you dig deeper. Start with the obvious: what has baby eaten? Is her tummy upset? Are there any rashes? Does baby look sick?

When do babies start teething?

- Baby will get cold-like symptoms just before they are cutting teeth, or they may be fussy for no other reason and cry more than normal. My obstetrician told me my son had a bad cold and wanted him to take medication, but all my children got their first teeth at four months. I have heard some get their teeth earlier.

I am not sure what to do when we get home.

- The best advice I can give for mum is to sleep every time baby sleeps, eat, feed baby and let everyone else around you do all other household chores. Learn to listen to your baby and go with your instincts. You will learn what baby needs quickly. Dads will get a lot of bonding time, especially after the first couple of weeks. The best thing dad can do is look after his wife. She will fall in love with you again for what you do to help her in the first couple of months.

Should I swaddle my baby?

- Your baby may love the freedom from the confined womb where he grew to capacity for nine months. On the other hand it may take some time for baby to learn that he is safe and okay not to be bundled. Follow his cues.

*Breathe and Believe.*
You *Can* Do It!

*"It's too bad babies don't come with a 'how-to' guide."*

*"We are made to do this work and it's not easy ... I would say that pain is part of the glory, or the tremendous mystery of life. And that if anything, it's a kind of privilege to stand so close to such an incredible miracle."*
**Simone in Klasson 2001**

*"Couples always seem to renovate or move when pregnant."*

# Induction and Augmentation Methods

Oxytocin, endorphins and adrenaline are three types of hormones that are released in your body naturally. Oxytocin is called the "love hormone" and is released while love-making. It helps start and stimulate contractions during labour and birth. The process helps dilate the cervix and move baby down and out, then helps to deliver the placenta and limits bleeding after the placenta. It is necessary in helping the breast with let down, or the milk ejection reflex for breast-feeding to occur. Together with prolactin, another hormone in the body, it makes us fall in love with our babies.

Low levels in labour can cause problems.

Endorphins are calming or pain-relieving hormones that we produce when we have pain or stress. We naturally release these in labour—some women have lower levels, but if you have higher than average levels this can help you cope with the pain of labour.

It is said that a dramatic drop in endorphin levels after birth is what causes the baby blues.

Adrenaline is the fight or flight hormone we produce to help ensure our survival. High levels produced in labour may make you feel fearful in labour, where lower levels may slow or stop it altogether.

You can help keep your hormones in check by staying calm, being confident and feeling comfortable where you labour. Have people that can keep you informed about what is happening, be prepared and have control over who is around you to ensure your privacy.

Try to avoid epidurals that can hamper your hormone levels, and be proactive about being in the best positions to labour.

When you go over your due date the care provider will want to encourage your body to start labour. They worry that as the placenta gets older it isn't working as efficiently and other complications can arise. Your care provider will assess how your cervix is to know the best way to start an induction method best suited for you. Care providers can tell if your cervix is ripe, which means it is softening and getting thinner, and the general positioning of the baby.

During pregnancy your cervix is closed, thick and posterior. When your body starts to get ready for labour, hormones are released and signal the start of the cervical changes. When you deliver your baby your cervix will be 10 cm dilated and paper thin, allowing baby's head to well apply itself into the pelvis and onto the cervix. When this natural progress hasn't started on its own, you may be induced.

Care providers send you for fetal non-stress testing. This tests the baby's heart rate and movements in a half-hour period; you lay on a bed with straps around your belly. Ultrasound checks the volume of amniotic fluid (the same procedure used to test due dates, an ultrasound is high frequency testing you can't hear but that projects an image onto a computer-type screen, and can see the amount of fluid in the amniotic sac). These tests ensure your baby's well-being, and help the care provider in deciding if they should start induction or wait for your body to naturally go into labour.

Acupressure or acupuncture are great ways to try to encourage labour to start and are done by a specialist. It is also done to augment your labour.

If the care providers believe that induction is in the best interest for your baby they may use a subtle technique like membranes sweep or stripping. They move their fingers around the inside lip of the cervix to stimulate it, and pull the membranes away from the mouth of the cervix. You may feel cramping and have some bloody discharge afterwards.

The next step after a few more days is to put a Cervidil or prostaglandin gel or tampon type insert onto the cervix. You are required to be in hospital for the procedure and they also want to monitor you and your baby. Sometimes women go into labor but not always on the first try. Most times you are sent home after the procedure is done. This procedure will help soften or ripen the cervix.

Induction and augmentation for labour and contractions can also be administered by I.V. when the care providers want to begin contractions or help them become stronger and closer together. You are admitted to hospital and given an I.V. attached to a drip with Oxytocin (pitocin). You are required to lie in bed and be monitored with belts around your belly. Oxytocin is increased and the contractions get stronger. Women generally ask for pain management. Gas will be the first relief offered and the epidural seems to be the most effective in giving total pain relief.

## Self-Induction Methods

There are some natural ways to try and induce or get things going if your cervix is already softening. Sex and lots of it can help. The semen contains prostaglandins and your orgasm releases Oxytocin and that can help the cervix to ripen or soften and put you into labour. The biggest issue may be getting both of you to want to do this.

Nipple stimulation is a great quick and easy way to start labour or if labour has stalled, may help to kick it back into gear. Cuddling and kissing will help to go a long way also.

Sometimes you can do things to start labour. A controversial one that I don't think anyone should try is drinking castor oil. You may put yourself in labour but it usually makes you throw up. Definitely not how I would want to labour.

Speculate on eating eggplant parmigiana. The oregano and basil in this dish have properties in them that may cause contractions, but there is no scientific research for this.

Evening Primrose Oil and Red Raspberry Leaf tea are two things that you can try in the last month of pregnancy and that are said to help ripen the cervix. Ask any health food or natural foods store where they stock these items.

## Placentas

When you go into labour you may lose the mucus plug and this is an indication that your body is getting ready for the birth. You can lose the plug anywhere from two weeks before or on the same day as labour starts. After the baby is born, the placenta is expelled usually within the hour after birth, and normally within minutes of birth. This is called the "afterbirth".

I am fascinated by placentas. This is the place where your baby has been growing for nine months and the amazing space that has nurtured her. The placenta is attached to the fetus by the umbilical cord and is attached to the inside of your uterus.

The placenta supplies the fetus with oxygen and nutrition from the mother and allows waste products and carbon dioxide to be released from the growing fetus. The umbilical cord is the baby's life line. It attaches at the stomach where the belly button will be. For those nine months, everything a baby needs to survive is sent through this cord.

The placenta is filled with rich blood vessels, and looks like a tree's root system on the outside. Inside, where baby lives, looks like rough calf's liver. In the cord there are three blood vessels; two are smaller arteries which carry blood to the placenta and the larger vein returns blood to the fetus, and this is covered with a clear membrane.

Inside, the placenta is filled with amniotic fluid. The fluid is a bit warmer than your body temperature and gives the baby a great place to grow and move around. It also protects baby from any outside bumps, or pressure from outside objects into your tummy.

After the baby is born, the cord is clamped, and some parents will ask specifically for the cord to stop pulsing first. Most times dad gets to cut the cord. The small bit of membrane dries over the next few days and falls off.

During pregnancy your baby moves around so much that she will entwine herself with the cord. During labour the baby's heart rate may lower with every contraction. This often will lead to concern by the care providers and you may end up having to have a Cesarean section. Other times the baby may be born with the cord wrapped around her throat several times, or as in this picture there was a perfect knot part way along the cord. This is common and cannot be prevented.

Some women like to take the placenta home for encapsulation, to plant in their gardens or to make art from.

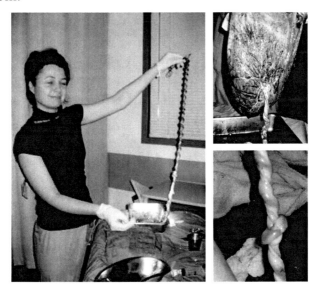

Pictured is my friend Tracy Kemp, a midwife, holding an exceptionally long cord. The cord was so thick that the knot had no effect on the baby's' heart beat, there was no decelerations in labour or birth.

*"We try to give a birthing woman freedom to find the right position for her own needs and comfort. Unfortunately, in our society we think of birthing as something done while lying down."*

**Michel Odent**

## Tidbits

I polled my clients and they came up with these tidbits of information. I asked them what worked for them when they came home with their new babies, and whether they garnered the advice through trial and error, or from a friend or family member. I hope some of it resonates with you.

Liam loved to go to sleep on daddy's chest so they did a lot of skin-to-skin. It was very soothing and reassuring. Baby-wearing rocks! Wearing baby in the Mei Tei and the wrap made my life easier and Liam loved it very much. It was great to bond with baby that way, especially after the Cesarean. Breast-feeding in a warm bath really, really helped! Massaging baby every evening made nights pretty peaceful—it works for rambunctious tots too. When Liam had little bouts of colic, we used the birthing ball to rock him and soothe him. Using the bicycle leg pumps also helped a lot in those cases.

**Elodie**

The only advice I ever found helpful (being a first-time mom, hearing a million different ways of doing things from various family members) was given to me by a friend. She said: "Just do what feels right." That advice pretty much made the only sense and I've stuck with it to this day.

**Lots of love, Danielle**

Although before Kaitlyn was born I had never even heard of baby-wearing, I became a huge fan when Kaitlyn came home. It felt so wonderful to have Kaitlyn in a wrap, napping away. And it was a great way for my husband to enjoy our newborn.

In the first few weeks, there were times when it felt like there was little I could do to console my new little bundle. But one night I started humming, and Kaitlyn calmed down so quickly. I realized that she loved to hear my voice, and found singing very soothing. I have a pretty average (perhaps worse than average) singing voice, but she loved it, and it was so incredible to connect with her and help her relax.

When your milk comes in, it can be quite uncomfortable. One of the more common recommendations is to put frozen cabbage in your bra. Well, the night my milk came in, I was desperate, so I sent my husband to the store for cabbage. There were two types: Savoy cabbage and purple cabbage. Well, the Savoy cabbage was more expensive, and apparently made my husband hungry, so he bought the purple cabbage for my swollen breasts. I am happy to report that the frozen cabbage was extremely helpful; however, the purple leaked all over our bed, all over our clothes, and all over my baby! We were both purple for days! My recommendation: splurge for the expensive cabbage.

Connect with the mummy network! It is amazing how helpful other mothers will be if you reach out. And there is nothing too graphic or embarrassing once you have been through childbirth.

Be open to trying different things to find out what works best for your child. We're told to put our babies on their backs to sleep but after one month of Brooke barely sleeping – two-hour stints at most and not falling asleep at night until 1:00 a.m. – I thought she was colic. Then for her naps I tried putting her on her stomach and she fell asleep quickly and for three to four hours. At six weeks I got brave enough to try her sleeping on her tummy at night and what a difference. Not only was there minimal crying at bedtime but she slept for five to six hours without a feeding and was a much happier, well-rested baby during the day. I was wrong thinking I had a difficult, colicky baby. She has a wonderful disposition and became the smiliest baby I'd ever seen!

I stalled the pushing stage because I believed it would hurt more, that was not the case. Also when we did the traditional three breaths per contraction I couldn't find my rhythm, but with my second baby we tried taking two breaths for each contraction and it worked extremely well.

**Shannon**

The hairdryer: by fluke, Lauren had read that to prevent diaper rash, use a hair dryer on the low setting on baby's bottom to ensure dryness. However when they dried baby's bottom she fell asleep. They now turn the hairdryer on every time their daughter isn't going to sleep. They even tried taping the sound, but it isn't as effective as the real sound.

P.S. Now Lauren can dry her hair as long as she wants and her baby will gently fall fast asleep.

**Lauren**

Tea made from fresh lemongrass really helped with breast milk production.

**My client received this information
from an African woman**

## A Single Mum's Birth Story – Anonymous

My client was a divorced woman who chose to have her second baby with the help of a sperm donor. She had a great team of fabulous friends; some of them have specialties that would enhance her birth experience. She knew she would need help when she got home. She designed the great schedule that I included in this book.

The best part was she knew what she *did not* want for this labour, specifically because of the result of her first birth experience. Unfortunately there had been some confusion with the doula and she didn't manage to make it to the birth, so mum had laboured all on her own. This time she was determined to change that and have the support and experience of a doula with her as it was her second and last child.

Mum wanted to hire a doula that would guarantee 100% she would attend the birth. I have never had any one explicitly ask that question, but I totally understood her concern and sympathized with her after she told me what had happened. I told her that I would definitely be there, providing I wasn't deathly ill.

Mum wanted this birth as natural as possible, which included no I.V.s and no needles! She was terrified of needles and was so worried that it might induce an asthma attack, which she knew could happen if she was stressed about her labour. So a calm birth would be essential.

She was also concerned about doctors. Over the years she found it a challenge to deal with them, which was her polite way of saying she had had a bad history with doctors.

In addition to hiring me, mum had rounded out her team with two good friends both because of their professional services: a massage therapist and an acupuncturist. They both had attended births in a professional capacity.

Mum was hoping that her baby would be born on her due date which was the same day as her beloved and recently passed away grandmother's birthday.

Six weeks before the due date mum had some swelling in her feet, and her blood pressure was starting to climb, so she had been asked if she would cut back on her work schedule. The doctor was also thinking of stripping / sweeping her membranes early to get labour started. Thankfully, this never happened.

*A month before the due date baby's head is very low in the pelvis. Mum is not sleeping more than one or two hours at a time as she simply can't get comfortable. There is more swelling in her feet. The doctor is talking about sweeping her membranes, again, so mum has booked off work. Mum is advised to stop taking Evening primrose and drinking Red raspberry tea as the doctor is wondering if this is contributing to these symptoms.*

*Two weeks before the due date, doctor checks her cervix and mum is 1-2 cm dilated and soft so she will put off induction for now. There is concern that her blood pressure is a bit high. A week later (one week before the due date) doctor sweeps her membranes. Mum is not sleeping very well, she is 2 cm dilated, her cervix is posterior and doctor wants to try Cervidil tomorrow morning to induce labour.*

---

*Evening Primrose is a natural oil high in prostaglandins that is used by many midwives to help soften and ripen the cervix to help with dilatation and help with the onset of labour. This is not recommended before 34 weeks.*

*Red raspberry tea is said to ready the uterus for labour, and make labour and birth easier and less painful. It has also been associated with relieving a lot of pregnancy complaints such as morning sickness and leg cramps. The tea can be frozen and taken during labour, similar to the Labour Aid. The tea is said to contain many minerals and is generally good for your health.*

*Please talk to your care provider when wanting to take these. Health food stores will have more extensive information on these and other teas that can be taken while pregnant.*

---

*8:00 a.m.: Mum arrives at the hospital with her friend (the designated driver) Jane. The induction method will be Cervidil, which is put on the cervix, and monitoring for mum begins. The doctor finally arrives to administer the Cervidil at 11:00 a.m. mum's cervix is almost totally effaced and 1-2 cm dilated. Also her cervix is high and posterior.*

*12:20 p.m.: I arrive at the hospital, partly because I am curious about how mum is really doing. It is hard not having telephone contact and she has been in the hospital for some time.*

*There have been tightenings in her stomach but no real contractions yet, and mum is content. She's a little tired from just hanging around the hospital all morning, but she is in very good spirits—it is, of course, going to be her daughter's birthday.*

*1:10 p.m.: I talk the nurses into allowing mum to get out of bed for the first time since arriving. Mum has a refreshing shower, which makes her feel much better. We start walking up and down corridors.*

*2:30 p.m.: The doctor comes in to check her cervix. Mum is 3 cm dilated. Doctor decides to break her water to increase the intensity and length of the contractions.*

*2:40 p.m.: Mum's other good friend Mary has been at work and we have had telephone contact for several hours. She is so worried that she won't make it to the hospital in time to help and that she'll miss the birth.*

*Mary finally arrives. Now Jane can go to attend her meeting in Vancouver. She waited for Mary to show up and is now worried she will miss the birth. She asks mum to please not have the baby until she gets back. These women are truly excited to help with the labour and birth, and it is very nice to see such support for mum.*

*4:15 p.m.:* Jane has come back from her meeting and now our little entourage has been walking with mum for quite a while, having lots of water and cranberry juice and sneaking crackers and cookies (the nurses would not allow mum to eat.) We decide to take a break from walking and put mum into the shower again.

*4:45 p.m.:* Mum is out of the shower; she is starving, and asks if she can eat. The dinner trays are being delivered, and the nurse finally agrees. (I am not sure about the mentality behind starving a labouring mum, but then I am not the clinical expert.) Mum gets hot tasteless broth and after adding salt and pepper declares it is just as bad. Mum finishes what little she can from the tray and goes to sit on the toilet. While there she has one big huge contraction that brings her to tears. There is lots of show and mucus in the toilet, and mum mentions the mild pressure in her bottom. We decide to carry on walking the halls.

*5:40 p.m.:* While walking, mum is having lots of strong, long contractions. They are making her stop and truly concentrate. There is a lot of bottom pressure. We try to distract mum by getting her to envision her cervix as a flower. She picks her favourite, a lotus flower, and we describe the blossom opening. We describe how beautiful it is when it opens, softly and gently. Mum has been clenching her body, and this technique works very effectively to help mum relax her body, especially in her bottom.

*5:15 p.m.:* Mum asks if she can be checked again, and after hearing she is 3.5 cm dilated, mum is not at all impressed.

*6:10 p.m.:* We decide a shower might be the best place for mum to relax and ease her contractions. If we had a tub that would surely be much better but at least we have a *great shower (I would love to see every labour and delivery room have both).*

*6:55 p.m.: Mum looks at us with big eyes and very sternly tells us she wants to push! Sometimes you just instinctually know what to do—I push the red button in the bathroom, and by the time mum is getting out of the shower we have a doctor and a room full of nurses.*

*We walk mum to the bed and get her settled. The doctor checks—the cervix is 10 cm dilated!*

*If by magic, Carol the acupuncturist arrives at the door. She comes close to mum and asks if she can use needles. Mum definitely wants anything that will help, so out come the needles. Carol is twirling them between her fingers and pushing them gently into ears and other parts of mum. We know that it's working because mum sighs and melts into the bed.*

*7:30 p.m.: Deb the massage therapist arrives. Mum has been pushing, along with direction from Mary, Jane and myself, and acupuncture from Carol. Now she is blessed with the wonderful hands of Deb who gives a professional massage. I am amazed that this petite woman has such powerful strength in her body. She contorts her body to get the perfect angle to give mum the best massage. Both of these women have attended birth before specifically for their professional specialties and are such assets to this birth.*

*8:10 p.m.: All day long the cervix has been posterior— the doctor checks progress and announces that this is now +2, which means it is no longer posterior and the head is quite low.*

*We have been trying several positions. I suggest hands and knees; we help move mum around and we immediately see a huge change in the effectiveness of the pushing.*

*8:25 p.m.: Sara emerges into the world and is placed skin-to-skin on mum's chest. A few minutes after Sara is being placed near mum's nipple and is looking to suckle. She is very clever and grasps on and sucks well.*

Mum had chosen a group of women that, except for the two friends, didn't know each other and we all worked in perfect unison to give mum the help she needed.

The other part of this amazing woman and her organizational skills was to have a schedule made up ahead of time. She emailed it to all her family and friends asking them if they could help in any way and to please fill it out and email it back. She co-ordinated one final schedule and sent it to everyone: the commitments made by each person where for cleaning, cooking, picking up and dropping the other child to and from school and play dates, even nap times for mum, and more.

It was her way of coping for the first few weeks as a single mum knowing she needed a commitment of support. She even had a different friend make the schedule for her!

I love that women can connect and work so well as a team.

# Afterword

IT IS OBVIOUS NOW; my passion for birth. I hope that I have given you food for thought and that you can journey through your birth knowing much more. I always wish an easy, short and uncomplicated labour for everyone.

I have only touched on a very small portion, of what a person having a baby will indeed need to know as this child grows. I sincerely hope that you and your new family, as small as it might stay or as large as it can grow, will have tons of joy and laughter. I wish that you will all be blessed with health.

Then somewhere after buying diapers, clothes and food for your growing brood, that you find enough abundance to treat yourself. I refer to both mum and dad, spend some money on yourself and remember why you wanted children and never forget why you are together.

*Love*

# Stay in Touch

IF YOU WANT TO STAY IN TOUCH with upcoming projects or follow my blog, I would love to hear from you. Please feel free to contact me. I will be writing more books in the future. I just may put you in my next book.

I have only talked about my small part of the world. I would love to travel. I would love to experience first-hand women labouring in different countries and learn your birth customs and your culture.

It has been a yearlong *labour* of love writing and publishing this book for you, and now I think I might plan to visit my favourite getaway and lay in the sun on a sandy beach.

Anything in life is possible. Remember to say I AM and envision where you want to be. One day you will wake up there.

### *Breathe and Believe!*

# About the Author

KIM A. TURTON IS A MOTHER, doula, private prenatal educator, Reiki Master, Director with the Constant Art Society, and authored a story in Doreen Virtue's book *The Healing Miracles of Archangel Raphael.* Her career as a professional birth coach started in 2001 when she established 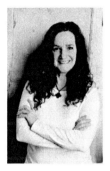 her business *My Doula.* This work allows her to follow her passion empowering women and assisting both them and their partners to birth their babies. Kim is kept busy working with private clients and the South Community Birth Program clients. She is very excited about birthing her new book.

Kim utilizes her extensive experience with an array of easy to difficult birth scenarios with all age groups of women and different cultures and backgrounds and her real life experience birthing four sons (a Cesarean section and three VBAC births) to bring compassion and understanding to birthing women. She draws on her personal and professional experience to excel at her career.

Kim has raised her wonderful boys into thriving young men. they have taught her much about life and given her immense joy and she believes they are her biggest accomplishments in life. She is a Reiki Master and lives a peaceful and spiritual life. With these teachings she guides people seeking a more balanced life. Kim spends her time writing, birthing and enjoying the outdoors where she lives in vibrant Vancouver, BC Canada, but she is partial to the warm waters and sandy beaches in Maui.

Kim has been a Director for the Constant Art Society for several years, a non-profit organization. Originally implemented as the Through Our Eyes Program in BC schools, the program was designed to connect youth to their community through photography and creative writing. The organization provides youth with opportunities to explore other mediums as outlets for self-expression.

Kim's goal is grace and dignity to every birthing woman, and peace and joy on this planet.

### *Breathe and Believe!*

Please visit these websites for more information on Kim Turton and her doula services.

**My Doula** - business website, describes what I offer as a doula, and my blog – *www.mydoula.ca*

**What Does a Doula Do?** - information page about the book – *www.whatdoesadouladdo.com*

**Inspired Authors Circle** and **Spiritual Authors Circle** are circles of authors that supported Kim Turton on her journey to publishing. Founded by Influence Publishing you can visit these websites to find out more about getting your own book written and published – 
*www.inspireabook.com*
*www.inspiredauthorscircle.com*
*www.spiritualauthorscircle.com*

CPSIA information can be obtained at www.ICGtesting.com

228479LV00005B/1/P

9 781907 498589